Take This Book to the

Dentist With You

OTHER PEOPLE'S MEDICAL SOCIETY BOOKS IN THIS SERIES

Take This Book to the Hospital With You

Take This Book to the Gynecologist With You

Take This Book to the Obstetrician With You

Take This Book to the Pediatrician With You

Take This Book

to the Dentist

With You

By
Charles B. Inlander
J. Lynne Dodson
and
Karla Morales

≡People's Medical Society®
Allentown, Pennsylvania

The People's Medical Society is a nonprofit consumer health organization dedicated to the principles of better, more responsive and less expensive medical care. Organized in 1983, the People's Medical Society puts previously unavailable medical information into the hands of consumers so that they can make informed decisions about their own health care.

Membership in the People's Medical Society is $20 a year and includes a subscription to the *People's Medical Society Newsletter.* For information, write to the People's Medical Society, 462 Walnut Street, Allentown, PA 18102, or call 610-770-1670.

This and other People's Medical Society publications are available for quantity purchase at discount. Contact the People's Medical Society for details.

Library of Congress Cataloging-in-Publication Data
Inlander, Charles B.
   Take this book to the dentist with you / by Charles B. Inlander,
J. Lynne Dodson, Karla Morales.
      p. cm.
   Includes index.
   ISBN 1-882606-27-2
      1. Dentistry—Popular works.   2. Dental care—Popular works.
3. Consumer education.   I. Dodson, J. Lynne.   II. Morales, Karla.
III. Title.
RK61.I55   1998
617.6—dc21   98-2958
                                                                  CIP

1 2 3 4 5 6 7 8 9 0
First printing, May 1998

To Lawrence A. Ross, D.D.S.,
with gratitude for his assistance with the preparation of this book
and for his years of dental care to J.L.D.

To Louis J. Morales, D.D.S.,
the best dentist and father anyone could have

CONTENTS

INTRODUCTION

Most of us dislike going to the dentist. And that's probably because we associate dentistry with pain. When I was a kid, as soon as the word "dentist" was spoken, someone within hearing range would utter an "ouch."

But dentistry has changed over the years to the extent that most dental work can be done almost painlessly. Plus, with the great advances in technology, most of us can expect a long life with our own natural teeth. Yet when something does go wrong, today's sophisticated dental techniques can usually fix it so that our teeth function almost as well as new ones.

But using dentistry and choosing a dentist are not always easy tasks. You might say it's a road dotted with cavities! No two dentists are the same. Even treatment options vary from dentist to dentist. And how do you choose between a general dentist and a specialist? When is one better than the other? Also, let's not forget cost. What do you do if you can't afford a $600 crown or thousands of dollars for an implant? Does Junior really need those braces? Then there are those controversial dental x-rays we hear so much about. Are they safe?

For more than a decade, we here at the People's Medical Society have been asked to write a book about dentistry. Consumers wanted to know how to choose a dentist, what to look for (and look out for). They've asked about the other people in the dental office, such as the hygienist and dental assistant. In recent years, we've been asked to address dental managed care programs and explain how they work and what a consumer should ask before joining.

Take This Book to the Dentist With You is our response to those thousands of requests. And we've done exhaustive research to help you choose and use a dentist. We believe we have covered everything you'll need to know to get the most from your dental encounters.

Take This Book to the Dentist With You is the latest in our series of "Take This Book With You" books. From *Take This Book to the Hospital With You* to *Take This Book to the Pediatrician With You,* this series has been enormously popular. Readers tell us what they like most about these books is the proconsumer, easy-to-read-and-understand style. Our goal is to help you better negotiate health care services.

We believe that your relationship with a health care practitioner should be a partnership. And while a dentist may be well trained and technically skilled in his or her art, *you* must ultimately make the decisions about what happens in your mouth. For that you need information. That is what we provide in the pages that follow.

We know there has never been a more comprehensive book written about dentistry for consumers. We have pored through the research, talked to the experts and listened to consumers in putting this book together.

So take this book to the dentist with you, and we're confident you'll get the highest level of care and best possible outcome.

CHARLES B. INLANDER
President
People's Medical Society

Take This Book to the
Dentist With You

We have tried to use male and female pronouns in an egalitarian manner throughout the book. Any imbalance in usage has been in the interest of readability.

Before You Go

ost of us associate dentists with the care of our teeth. We've undergone more than our share of oral examinations, complete with fairly regularly scheduled x-rays. We've probably had a few silver fillings, known as amalgams, and perhaps even a crown, a gold or ceramic covering for a fractured or seriously decayed tooth.

But the fact is that modern dentistry covers much more than "fixing teeth." True, about half of all dental treatment relates to caries—better known to most of us as tooth decay—but during an oral examination, your dentist looks closely at your gums for signs of infection or other gum disease. Dentists are able to diagnose, treat and prevent diseases of the tongue, lining of your cheeks (mucosa), palate and jawbones, as well as the teeth and gums, and may spot the first signs of oral cancer. As we describe later, some dental specialists perform surgery to correct deformities in, or injuries to, the mouth or jaw. Other specialists apply braces to correct tooth alignment.

Modern dentistry has also expanded its knowledge of many topics, including anesthesia and other pain control, anatomy of the mouth, and surgical techniques. Unfortunately, though, great areas of knowledge lay untapped. Here's a case in point.

More than 20 years ago, research began on variations in medical practices, evaluating rates of use of various procedures and initiating considerable research on the outcome and effectiveness of recommended treatments. In dentistry, however, little similar research has been carried out. As a result, neither consumers nor dentists can know which treatment is best in a given situation. In 1995, University of North Carolina professors James D. Bader, D.D.S., M.P.H., and Daniel A. Shugars, D.D.S., Ph.D., M.P.H., reported in the *Journal of Public Health Dentistry* on their comprehensive review of the few studies that had been done on dentists' clinical treatment decisions. Their conclusion? Variation in dentists' clinical decisions was widespread. Here are some of the areas of disagreement and inconsistency that Bader and Shugars reported.

- In a county in the South, the proportion of crown applications versus fillings for large cavities was three times greater than elsewhere in the survey.

- When 700 North Carolina dentists taking part in a mailed questionnaire survey reviewed photographs of several teeth with worn spots or chips on the outer surface, 46 percent indicated they would work to restore the damaged teeth, while 47 percent said they would leave the teeth as they were. The remaining 7 percent would provide another treatment such as adjusting the patient's bite.

- A 1984 study asked more than 300 Washington State dentists to prepare treatment plans based on written descriptions of five elderly patients. The researchers found "substantial unexplained variation" in the plans for any given patient.

So what's a consumer to do? Unfortunately, as Bader and Shugars point out, so little information describing outcomes of dental treatment is available that "the appropriateness of much of dental care cannot be assessed." Thus, the wise dental consumer must ask questions, get a second and even third opinion before deciding on major treatments and evaluate the care based on previous experience, personal needs and a measure of gut feeling.

Without agreement on what's "best" in dental care, you must also work to find a dentist you can trust—one who involves you in planning your care, recognizes your desire to make truly informed decisions and works with you to keep your teeth without losing your life savings. Your search for such a dentist begins with asking questions, getting several opinions and using your own knowledge, long before you actually visit a dentist.

CHOOSING YOUR DENTIST

Dentistry is a very up-close and personal service. You sit just inches away from the dentist with his fingers in your mouth for what may seem like an eternity. You may be fearful or anxious.

The first step in finding a dentist who has your health and comfort in mind is to put together a list of possible candidates.

Unfortunately, your choices may be limited by your geographic location. In 1993, there were at least 1,000 areas within the country that had been designated "dental health professional shortage areas," including nearly 200 predominantly rural counties with no general or pediatric dentists at all. Only about 6 percent of the approximately 166,000 practicing dentists live in the western mountain region, comprised of Idaho, Montana, Wyoming, Nevada, Utah, Colorado, New Mexico and Arizona. Yet 18 percent practice in the three mid-Atlantic states of New York, Pennsylvania and New Jersey. California alone has 13 percent. If you live in an area with few dentists, you may have to be more creative and persistent in your search for a competent dentist. Use every one of the sources described below if necessary. But even if your choices are limited, take the time to carefully evaluate the dentist, the staff and the office.

As a starting point, you can refer to these resources for names of possible candidates.

■ *American Dental Directory,* an annual publication of the American Dental Association (ADA) that can be found in the reference section of many larger libraries. This directory lists ADA-member dentists (about 75 percent of all actively practicing dentists) with their educational backgrounds, certifications and office addresses. The American Dental Association does not provide telephone referrals, but instead directs callers to their local dental societies.

■ Your local dental society, listed in the telephone directory, which can give you the names and telephone numbers of member dentists who are currently taking new patients. The society may also provide information on training and specialty certification. In an emergency, many societies maintain a list of dentists who have agreed to be on call on a rotating basis to provide care.

- Your dental managed care plan administrator. If you are covered by a dental health maintenance organization, preferred provider organization or other managed care plan, the plan maintains a list of participating dentists from which to choose, along with their education credentials, certifications and basic office information.

Your Options in Dental Plans

The availability of dental plans and dental benefits is a relatively new development for both dentists and consumers. Historically, dentistry was a "cash" business—meaning that you went to the dentist, received a service and paid the fee on your way out. You selected the dentist of your choice and had the freedom to either return for further care or change dentists as you pleased. Very few consumers had any type of dental coverage and even fewer companies offered dental coverage to their employees.

According to a recent survey conducted by *Human Resource Executive,* however, the number of businesses offering dental benefits to their employees has reached 91 percent. Of the companies offering benefits, 38 percent offer a managed care plan.

There are four basic types of dental plans: direct reimbursement, indemnity insurance, dental preferred provider organization (PPO) and dental health maintenance organization (HMO). Any or all of these plans may have a managed care component that requires prior approval for some services.

- *Direct reimbursement plans.* These plans are essentially cash plans because when you receive a service, you pay the dentist out of pocket and then are reimbursed by your employer or the plan's administrator. Fees are usually discounted and your

continued

reimbursement is based on a percentage of those fees. You may incur either a copayment per service or a maximum out-of-pocket expense.

- **Indemnity insurance.** The concept behind this type of plan is probably familiar to you since most insurance plans for the past 50 years have been based on it. In a nutshell, indemnity plans reimburse dentists according to a fee schedule or an allowance for some specialized services (such as crowns, braces and certain types of fillings). In order to receive a covered service, you must select a "participating" dentist—meaning that the dentist has a contract with the insurance company and agrees to accept the fee as payment in full.

- **Dental preferred provider organization.** This type of plan introduces, for the first time, elements that not only affect the way dentists are selected, but also may influence treatment options. In a dental PPO, a group of dentists agree to discount their fees in return for patients being directed to them for all dental services. The thinking here is that each dentist in the group will gain additional patients, thereby increasing volume and eventually the bottom line.

   In reality, if you're in a dental PPO, you may find your choice of dentist severely restricted, and you may even need to change dentists if you want full coverage from the plan. While influencing treatment decisions is not a major goal of the dental PPO, there is still the concern that dentists may be reluctant to provide all treatment options if they feel the discounted fee is too low.

- **Dental health maintenance organization.** The dental HMO is the most restrictive plan in terms of your selection of dentists. Dental HMOs have contracts with dentists to provide the care and services you require in exchange for a fixed monthly fee. This is called a capitation fee, and it literally means "paid on each head" for every member of the HMO. Typically,

continued

all of your care is covered 100 percent, although there may be a small copayment ranging from $5 to $10 for each visit.

In order to receive services, you must use a dentist in the HMO; if you go outside the plan, there is no coverage. Prior approval for certain types of dental services (crowns, braces and oral surgery) may also be required by the HMO.

For consumers, concerns must center on the quality of care and the competence of the plan's dentists. The few studies that have compared managed care with traditional (fee-for-service) dentistry have shown no clear-cut quality differences. A 1990 study, for example, found that both fee-for-service and capitation programs were inconsistent in providing good dental care. A study of care for children in England and Scotland found that dentists in managed care plans provided more preventive care but let cavities get to a later stage of development before filling than did fee-for-service dentists.

Managed care dental plans generally provide basic information about the dentists in their plans. This probably includes education, specialty, any specialty certification and years in practice. While such information may be helpful, you still need to become actively involved in selecting your dentist.

Some managed care plans actually encourage meetings between their dentists and prospective members. And if you aren't satisfied with your first choice, make sure you know and understand the procedure for changing dentists.

■ Nearby dental schools, which may be able to provide the names of faculty members who maintain private practices, and hospitals with in-patient dental services, which may be able to give you the name of dentists with admitting privileges to the hospital (meaning they can send their patients there and care for them while they are hospitalized)

■ Your physician, especially if you have a medical condition such as diabetes that could complicate your dental care

■ Dental referral services, which are commercial agencies that provide referrals to dentists who pay for the service. Your choices will be restricted to dentists who participate, and the information you receive will be general, such as training, years in practice and office location. You can be assured, however, that the referred dentist is taking new patients. These services have toll-free numbers; you can find them in the toll-free telephone directory or your local Yellow Pages, or by calling the toll-free directory assistance line at 800-555-1212.

■ Newspaper advertisements, which historically merely announced a new practice, but which in recent years appear also for established practices. One type, the "advertorial," looks like an article and provides information on dental health. The dentist's name, office location and telephone number are usually given, which is one of the signals distinguishing this advertisement from a true newspaper article. As a resource, newspaper advertisements tell you a dentist is accepting new patients, but they don't tell you why. The dentist may have recently graduated from dental school, moved to the area for the climate or relocated from another state after losing his license. You will have to find out more before entrusting your care to this dentist.

■ Yellow Page advertisements, which are paid for by the dentist. As with newspaper advertisements, dentists who advertise in the Yellow Pages signal their willingness to accept new patients. Because the information in the advertisement is provided by the dentist, you will need to verify all claims by careful questioning.

■ Friends, relatives and work associates, who are likely to be able to give you information on a dentist's manner, policies and items such as office hours and availability of parking. This source may be less reliable in discussing the dentist's education or professional competence.

If you'll need a new dentist because of a planned relocation, ask your present dentist for a referral. Many have informal networks through school or affiliations with professional organizations. If your present dentist is retiring, he will also give you a referral to another local dentist. In either situation, you will still want to carry out your own evaluation, based on the information in the following sections. At least you'll have a head start on your list of candidates.

Questions to Ask Yourself

Once you have the names and telephone numbers of several dentists, you're ready to begin your evaluation. Start first, though, by asking yourself several questions. Your answers can help you focus on just what it is that you need and want from your dentist.

1. **Do I want "one-stop" shopping with a general dentist who can provide most of my care or a specialist to handle a specific problem?**

Dentistry is still dominated by generalists, rather than specialists. About eight in 10 dentists have trained as general practitioners. They offer preventive care such as cleanings, as well as treatments ranging from fillings to surgical removal of third molars, your wisdom teeth.

Unlike medical specialists, there are many fewer dental specialists, and referrals to designated specialists are much less common. Some procedures, such as orthodontics (correction of bite problems, for example with braces), are performed only by specialists. Others, such as periodontics (gum disease therapy), may be performed by a general dentist unless there are complications such as major infection, in which case you would be referred to a periodontist. You'll find more about specialists later in this chapter.

Are there any firm guidelines for when specialty care is preferred over general care, or vice versa? Not much research has been done comparing the care given by specialists versus that of general dentists. In 1994, however, a report in the *Journal of Oral and Maxillofacial Surgery* described differences in recommendations for a patient with four wisdom teeth that had not erupted above the gum line. Eighty percent of oral surgeons who reviewed the case recommended surgery, whereas only 43 percent of the general dentists advised surgery.

The American Dental Association Code of Ethics requires certified specialists to practice their specialty exclusively, so even if you need a specialist for a specific condition, you will also need to have a general dentist for ongoing care.

2. **Do I want a solo practitioner or a group of dentists?**

More than two out of three dentists are solo practitioners, so finding one may be easier than locating a group practice. The typical solo practice includes the dentist and one or more chairside assistants. These assistants prepare the dental instruments, mix materials used in fillings and other procedures and work alongside the dentist in caring for patients. About 60 percent of solo dentists also employ one or more dental hygienists, who are trained and licensed to carry out basic examinations, cleanings, x-ray procedures and patient education. You'll find more about the training and responsibilities of both assistants and hygienists later in this chapter.

Dental group practices tend to be small, with only two to three dentists on average. Only about 12 percent of private practice dentists work in groups with three or more dentists. Group practices are likely, however, to have larger staffs than solo dentists, with nine of 10 groups having two or more chairside assistants and seven of 10 having at least one dental hygienist.

Both practice types have potential advantages and disadvantages that may be important to you. With only one dentist and a small staff, the solo practice encourages a close dentist-patient relationship. You can't be shuffled from dentist to dentist as might happen in a group.

The very qualities that make for a close relationship, however, also raise the potential for problems. With only one dentist, office hours may not be as convenient as you would like, nor may the office schedule be always able to accommodate yours. When the dentist is away or otherwise unavailable, your care must come from someone outside the practice whom you have never met. There are no professional colleagues whom your dentist can regularly consult, learn from or be challenged by.

If you are willing to be seen by any of the dentists in a group, you're likely to find evening and weekend hours and 24-hour emergency coverage. In the best-run groups, the staff members share with each other what they learn from journals and conferences, helping to keep everyone current. Your dentist can call on a second pair of hands or eyes in case of an emergency or before making a recommendation. If you find a group that includes both general dentists and one or more specialists, you can stay with the same group for all your care.

On the other hand, the larger staff means you have more credentials and practice habits to evaluate and monitor. You must ask about the background of each dentist, hygienist and assistant before her hand goes into your mouth or he prepares to take x-rays.

You may find this task made more difficult by staff turnover. New dental graduates are joining groups as salaried dentists—not as part owners of the practice—in ever-increasing numbers. According to the American Association of Dental Schools, nearly one-third of seniors plan to take salaried jobs on graduation. Many will work long enough to pay off education loans and raise capital before leaving to open their own practices.

3. Do I want a dentist who outlines a treatment plan with options from which to choose or one who makes the treatment decisions for me?

In a major review in the *Journal of Dental Education* of what is currently known about dental treatment variations and outcomes, University of North Carolina professors James D. Bader and Daniel A. Shugars wrote, "Most of dentistry's day-to-day procedures are rendered in the absence of comprehensive knowledge of their expected results." In other words, even the dentist probably doesn't know what the long-term effects of treatment are. Bader and Shugars assert that dentists are poorly prepared to assess the validity of studies or to interpret statements of risk in selecting treatment alternatives.

Charles G. Widmer, D.D.S., and colleagues at Emory University's Dental Research Center agree. In a *California Dental Association Journal* article, they wrote, "Most dentists are not given courses on statistics and scientific methodology in dental school," leaving dentists unprepared to critically evaluate scientific research on treatments and other topics.

Despite these potential shortcomings, in order to give truly informed consent, you should be given a treatment plan that outlines the following: treatment alternatives, advantages and disadvantages of each alternative, risks of each, costs of each and the likely result of doing nothing.

4. Do I want a dentist who is prevention oriented and who provides information about steps I can take at home to lessen the need for dental therapy?

Historically, dental education and licensing procedures emphasized technical skill in diagnosis and treatment. Dentists were evaluated on how well they filled a tooth or fitted a crown.

Within the past two decades, however, the consumer wellness focus has made itself felt within dentistry. Several schools have reorganized the patient-care portion of their training so that each student has an assigned group of patients to care for throughout the program. This patient-focused care more closely simulates private practice than did the previous system of assigning a patient on a first-come, first-served basis to any available student at every visit. The new system provides greater continuity of care and offers more opportunities for the student to apply prevention techniques, such as cleaning teeth and applying fluoride to prevent decay, and to give advice on at-home oral care.

Fluoride treatments, sealants and other developments that help prevent decay play a role in encouraging prevention efforts. As we detail later in this book, the 50-year history of water fluoridation, fluoride toothpastes and direct fluoride application to children's teeth has been a major factor in decreasing levels of tooth decay, especially on the vertical (rather than chewing) surfaces of teeth. Sealants have a shorter history, but these plastic coatings appear to be effective when applied to the horizontal (chewing) surfaces of molars (the large back teeth).

Managed care is a third factor encouraging preventive dentistry. Health maintenance organizations, preferred provider organizations and other types of managed care plans pay for care that is provided by a preapproved list of dentists. These plans pay for preventive measures such as regular examinations and cleanings, thus encouraging patients to schedule them and dentists to perform them.

One signal that a practice is prevention oriented is the presence of a dental hygienist on staff. Your dentist shows his concern for prevention by providing brochures from the American Dental Association and other health organizations; health-oriented magazines; and models, videotapes and other oral hygiene training tools for children and adults.

5. Do I have a medical condition that could affect my oral health or that requires special monitoring during dental care?

If you have diabetes, hemophilia, a transplanted organ, heart disease, asthma or any other chronic health condition, you are most likely aware of the complications that can arise during even relatively minor dental procedures (see chapter 6).

For now, make sure to note any allergies, chronic conditions or recent illnesses and ask prospective dentists about their experience in caring for patients with similar conditions. According to studies by the Eastman Dental Center in Rochester, New York, dentists who completed an additional year of training after their four years of dental school (called a postdoctoral general dentistry program), instead of entering practice immediately on graduation, are more likely to treat patients with serious medical conditions or handicaps, to spend more time on the physical examination of their patients and to use medical laboratories more often.

6. Do I have a strong preference for a dentist who is young versus old or female versus male?

While finding someone who is competent, willing to involve you in care decisions and concerned for your comfort is probably uppermost in your mind, you may have age or gender criteria that you want to consider. No recent studies have analyzed age- and gender-based differences in care, but we can tell you that only about 13 percent of actively practicing dentists are women.

7. Are there special circumstances in my lifestyle that may affect my choice of dentist?

For instance, if your daily schedule is a whirl of work, family and community obligations, fitting dental appointments into your date book is one more challenge. Take a moment, when selecting your dentist, to consider some factors that could make scheduling a bit easier. For example, do you want a dental office that is:

- Accessible from bus or other mass transportation?
- Open early mornings, evenings and/or Saturdays?
- Flexible about last-minute cancellations?
- Located within a specified distance from your home or workplace?

8. How do I plan to pay for care? Do I have access to dental insurance? What are its provisions for coverage? If I am a member of an HMO or other managed care plan, how does my choice of dentist affect coverage?

We discuss the financial aspects of dental care in detail in chapter 8; however, we can say here that finances can and often do play a role in your choice of dentist. Approximately 60 percent of Americans age two and older are not covered by dental insurance or government assistance programs such as Medicaid. If you are uninsured or have very limited coverage, you will need to plan for paying for your care. This may mean finding a dentist who is willing to be paid in installments or by credit card.

Further, even if you are covered by dental insurance, you cannot assume that all dentists or procedures are included. Read your policy and know its primary features. If a dentist you are considering does not accept your insurance plan, you will have to pay the bill in full and then submit your claim for payment—which will probably not be the full amount.

If you participate in one of the several types of managed care plans, your choice of dentist may be restricted. The traditional HMO provides coverage as long as you use a dentist within the HMO network. In order to keep members in competitive markets, however, some HMOs now allow patients to receive care from dentists outside the network, but the patient pays a greater portion of the fees out of pocket. Preferred provider organizations offer a list of dentists from which to choose who have agreed to provide care either at a discounted price or with you paying a portion of the fee (copayment). If you choose a nonparticipating dentist, you pay the full charges for your treatment.

Of course, in the best of all worlds, financial considerations should not play a role in your choice of a dentist or your plans for treatment. In reality, the better informed you are about your eligibility for coverage, the better able you will be to maximize your benefits to get the care you need.

9. **If I changed dentists in the past, why did I do so? What will I want the new dentist to do differently?**

Once you have established the various factors that are important to you, you can begin to evaluate the prospective dentists you have identified.

Questions to Ask the Dental Receptionist

You'll save time and money if you ask some questions on the telephone first, most of which can be answered by the receptionist. These questions are discussed below and included on the Dentist Information Worksheet (see Appendix). Make a copy and have it in front of you when you conduct both your initial telephone screening interview and your in-person visit. Attach each dentist's business card after your visit for future use. Once you have completed the worksheet, you are in a better position to compare dentists, giving priority to the answers to those questions that are most important to you.

When you call, explain that you are a potential new patient and ask:

1. Is the dentist taking new patients? If not, is there a waiting list? How long is it?

2. Does the dentist schedule get-acquainted visits? If yes, how much time is available? How much does such a visit cost?

Plan to schedule a visit during which no procedures will be done; in fact, you don't even have to sit in the dental chair. A get-acquainted visit gives you the opportunity to meet the dentist and staff, tour the office and get an overall impression *before* anyone pokes fingers in your mouth.

A face-to-face approach—similar to the way that dental care is delivered—is really the only way to fully evaluate the dentist's answers to your questions. You can detect signs of unease or defensiveness and observe how well the staff seems to work together. Of course, it's also the only way to see the condition of the instruments and equipment to be used in your care.

Get-acquainted visits are likely to be more common in urban areas. There, competition for patients may be intense, and dentists find that get-acquainted visits are an effective marketing technique. Even if a dentist doesn't routinely offer one, he may agree to if prompted, so be sure to ask. And if the receptionist says no, suggest that she confirm this with the dentist.

You may have only 15 minutes, so take the Dentist Information Worksheet (see Appendix) and any additional written questions with you to guide the interview. Expect to pay for the visit, as it will not be covered by insurance.

3. Does the dentist limit the practice to a specialty? If so, is he board certified?

As we have indicated, specialization is much less common in dentistry than in medicine, with fewer than 20 percent of dentists practicing a specialty. The American Dental Association recognizes eight specialties:

■ *Endodontics.* Endodontists treat the inside of the teeth, primarily the soft pulp. Most commonly, they perform root canal treatment, including cleansing, sterilizing and filling the canal. While general dentists will often perform uncomplicated root canal therapy, a specialist is likely to carry out the procedure if the root is abscessed or the bone or other structures around the tooth could cause complications. If you need a crown placed on the tooth after the root canal, the endodontist will probably refer you to your general dentist who can complete the procedure.

■ *Oral and maxillofacial surgery.* These specialists extract teeth, as well as perform surgery on the mouth, jaws, chin and related muscles. While simple extractions can be performed by your general dentist, an oral surgeon will usually be called in if you have a medical condition that could complicate the surgery, a wisdom tooth that is impacted (imbedded in the bone under the gum) or a need for another specialized procedure. Jaw reconstruction, certain types of cosmetic facial surgery and similar procedures requiring surgical skill are also commonly performed by these specialists.

■ *Oral pathology.* Oral pathologists study tissue from the mouth and teeth to diagnose disease and recommend therapy. They commonly work in hospitals, laboratories and other institutions.

■ *Orthodontics.* Orthodontists correct malocclusion (misalignment of teeth) by applying braces to the teeth to slowly move them into the correct position. In the past, most of their patients were children and teenagers, but increasing numbers of adults are undergoing the procedure. Your general dentist can refer you to an orthodontist or you can choose your own. The course of treatment can last up to two years (or more in adults), is expensive and is seldom fully covered by insurance, so look for an orthodontist with both a compatible personality and financial flexibility.

■ *Pediatric dentistry.* Also known as pedodontics, this specialty treats children's teeth. Pediatric dental training involves not only medical and dental issues, but also child psychology and development. Thus, children with behavioral problems that would prevent them from sitting quietly in a dental chair or children with disabilities or unusual dental problems are most likely to be referred to this specialist.

■ **Periodontics.** These specialists treat the gums and supporting bone around your teeth. They are most commonly called in to perform gum surgery, such as recontouring, tightening or grafting gum tissue.

■ **Prosthodontics.** Prosthodontists replace all or part of damaged or missing teeth with artificial teeth: caps, bridges and dentures. While general dentists also perform these procedures, these specialists care for the difficult cases beyond the scope of most general dentists' training or experience.

■ **Public health dentistry.** These specialists set up community dental screenings and treatment programs, monitor trends in dental disease and carry out educational programs for dentists and the community at large.

As we describe in greater detail in the next section, the American Dental Association Code of Ethics specifies that dentists who promote themselves as specialists must have completed additional education beyond the four years of dental school and practice exclusively in their specialty. Sixteen states issue a separate license to specialists, who are also required to have a general dentistry license: Alaska, Arkansas, Idaho, Illinois, Kansas, Kentucky, Michigan, Minnesota, Mississippi, Missouri, Nevada, Oklahoma, Oregon, South Carolina, Tennessee and West Virginia.

While dental specialists are required to get a separate license in these states, they are not required to obtain board certification in any state. In fact, board certification is an additional step that only about one in three dental specialists takes. Each specialty has a national board, monitored by the Council on Dental Education of the American Dental Association. Dentists who have completed their advanced education and worked in their specialty for a specified number of years (this varies with the specialty—see page 45) can apply to take the certification examination. On successful completion, they become board certified.

Board certification is not an assurance of quality care. No studies have been carried out comparing certified and noncertified specialists. Certification does demonstrate that the dentist knew how to perform the procedures of his specialty at a specific moment and was willing to have that knowledge tested by an independent body. Certification also reflects the dentist's interest in education beyond basic dental training.

For further information, contact:

American Dental Association
211 E. Chicago Ave.
Chicago, IL 60611
312-440-2500

4. Who performs basic teeth cleaning—the dentist or a hygienist? If the hygienist, will the dentist do this if I request it?

As we've mentioned, most dentists practice without other dentists but not without staff. Hygienists work full- or part-time in 63 percent of dental offices. Some experts argue that because their education focuses on preventive techniques such as cleanings, dental hygienists are actually better trained than dentists to carry out these procedures.

Nevertheless, if you want the dentist to carry out all procedures on your mouth, say so up front. Don't wait until you're lying back in the dental chair.

5. What are the office hours? Are exceptions made for emergencies?

6. Does the dentist have a time set aside to receive and return patient telephone calls?

7. Who covers for the dentist when he is ill or on vacation?

Dentists who practice with a partner or in a larger group of dentists can usually rely on these colleagues to care for their patients during an absence. However, the majority of dentists practice solo and so must arrange for another dentist to provide emergency care when they are away. You will want to assure yourself that the covering dentist is as qualified as your permanent dentist. Ideally, your dentist selected him based on knowledge of his work and satisfaction of his patients. However, the selection could also have been influenced by family or school ties or simple expediency. Evaluate the covering dentist for yourself.

8. Does the dentist accept my dental insurance?

9. Does the dentist have a published fee schedule?

The availability of a printed fee schedule, while uncommon, will be the easiest way to compare fees among your prospective dentists. If a fee schedule is not available, ask for the fee for two basic procedures: for example, an annual oral examination without x-rays and an amalgam restoration (a silver filling) on one surface of a permanent tooth.

Your choice of dentist should not be made exclusively on the basis of the "lowest bidder." Nevertheless, the chances are high that you will pay at least a portion of the charges from your own pocket, so you will probably want to consider fees as one factor in your overall decision-making process.

THE GET-ACQUAINTED VISIT

You're now ready for the all-important on-site visit. You will find it worth both the time and money to talk with the dentist and staff without the anxiety of a pending examination or procedure. The visit gives you an opportunity to note not only answers to your questions, but also your own impressions and feelings about the dentist's overall demeanor and openness, qualities that can be difficult to discern over the telephone. You can observe the interplay between the dentist and his staff and between them and other patients.

The very act of scheduling a get-acquainted visit signals to the dentist and staff that you are an alert dental consumer. From the beginning, you identify yourself not as the patient submitting to whatever the dentist mandates, but as an informed person who will evaluate and choose from among options. If you have been a fearful dental patient in the past, you may also find that taking control and insisting on information allay many fears.

Bring a copy of the Dentist Information Worksheet (see Appendix) with you to guide your questioning and allow efficient note taking. Most questions need only brief answers and should be immediately answerable. You have a right to ask these questions. Note if the dentist becomes defensive, vague or nervous when answering.

Because most dentistry is performed in private offices with little or no oversight by government or accrediting agencies, your observations are critical. Focus on the setting, equipment and procedures, as well as the staff. Chapter 2 describes key features to look for in a well-run dental office, including emergency preparedness, infection control measures and x-ray safety. Observe the following:

1. Is the reception area clean, well-lit and large enough to accommodate waiting patients and their families?

2. Do people seem to wait a long time?

3. Are you greeted promptly?

4. Are you seen on time?

5. Are current health-related reading materials available?

As you sit down with the dentist, confirm any of the answers given earlier by the receptionist about which you have doubts. In addition, this is the time to ask about the dentist's training, experience and, perhaps most important, philosophy of care, with questions such as:

1. When and where did you receive your dental training?

2. Did you complete a general dentistry residency (see page 44)?

3. How long have you been in practice? Have you ever practiced in another state?

4. When does your current license to practice expire? Have you ever had your license suspended or revoked in this state or elsewhere?

5. What procedures do you commonly perform?
   Beware of the dentist who answers "Everything" to this last question. While specialization is much less common in dentistry than in medicine, you want to be wary of a general dentist who claims to commonly perform all procedures from fillings to oral surgery. Neither the dentist nor his assistants can keep their skills sharpened by carrying out an occasional surgery. Practice does make perfect.

6. Have you had special training to carry out newer procedures such as implants? If so, how long was it and where did you receive it?
   A lecture during a dental conference hardly constitutes training.

7. How often do you and your staff attend conferences and continuing education workshops?

8. Is your dental assistant certified (see page 47)?

9. Who performs x-ray examinations? If it's someone other than the dentist, has she received formal training (see page 66)?

10. Do you provide a written treatment plan? Does it include fees?

MAKING YOUR CHOICE

Once you have visited all of your potential dentists, review your notes and the checklist.

1. Does one dentist stand out in terms of his willingness to answer your questions?

2. Do you sense a better relationship is possible with one dentist versus the others?

3. Does one dentist's philosophy of dental care match yours better than the others?

4. Does one dentist meet all or most of the criteria that are most important to you such as evening appointments, acceptance of your insurance or participation in a group practice?

5. Did one dentist's staff make a better impression than the others?

If the answer to these questions is yes, you have cleared a major hurdle in establishing a satisfactory dentist-consumer relationship. It is a relationship based on an exchange of information, informed decision-making and mutual concern for your dental health. You may even enjoy going to the dentist!

Changing Dentists

Despite your care in selecting a dentist, you may at some point feel that a change may be necessary—or you may be forced by an employer switching to a dental managed care plan. For the dentist-consumer relationship to work, you must be able to trust in his work (not blindly, though) and feel that your best interests are being served. What are some of the circumstances that may signal a need to change dentists?

- The dentist takes telephone calls and otherwise fails to give you undivided attention during treatment.
- The dentist doesn't listen when you describe symptoms or concerns.
- The dentist is repeatedly behind schedule and his staff doesn't call ahead to suggest rescheduling.
- The dentist fails to describe your problem and suggest a treatment plan, including fees and the likely results of not undergoing treatment, so that you can make an informed decision regarding care.
- The dentist doesn't answer your questions or responds in a manner that you are unable to understand.
- The dentist is offended by your request for a second opinion for a major procedure.
- The office and equipment have become shabby or dirty or otherwise indicate a decline in standards.
- The dentist is hard to reach, fails to return telephone calls and/or doesn't arrange for office coverage during absences.
- You feel uncomfortable by remarks or behavior on the part of the dentist or a staff member.

These are just a few of the scenarios that may start you thinking about a change. Of course, there are other personal concerns—you may wish to find a dentist closer to your home or place of employment, or one whose office hours accommodate your work schedule and so on. If you have had a previously satisfactory relationship with your dentist, you may want to discuss your current concerns before actually making a change. The dentist may appreciate learning about problems with the staff, for example, and will initiate changes that enable you to stay with him.

If the breach is a serious one—you have been injured by the dentist's work, for instance—you may want to ask the local dental society for a peer review or grievance-resolution hearing (make sure that your dentist is a member of the local society) or file a formal complaint with your state dental licensing board.

According to the American Dental Association, "Every dental society has established a system to resolve the occasional disagreement about dental treatment that a patient and a dentist have not been able to resolve themselves. A peer review committee consists of dentists (and

sometimes laypersons) who volunteer their time and expertise to consider questions about the appropriateness or quality of care or, in certain
circumstances, about the fees charged for dental treatment."

After the written request for review is submitted to the state or local
dental society, the request is reviewed for completeness and referred to
an appropriate committee. A mediator—a member of the committee—
contacts all parties and attempts to reconcile the problem. There is also
an appeal process in the event that, after mediation, any of the parties
is not satisfied with the decision. Contact the American Dental Association (211 E. Chicago Ave., Chicago, IL 60611; 312-440-2500) or
your local dental society for further details about dentistry's dispute-
resolution program.

INSIDE DENTISTRY

A studied evaluation process is an important first step to ensure many
years of good dental care. But before you lay back in that dental chair,
let's look at what your new dentist had to do to be able to sit alongside you.

The Making of a Dentist

There are currently 55 dental schools in the United States. Applicants
must have completed at least two years of college (74 percent of students
entering in 1994 had a bachelor's degree and 5 percent had master's degrees or higher). They must also take the Dental Admission Test, a standardized test for all schools, and submit letters of recommendation.

The dental school program is four years long. During the first two
years, students study:
- Biology as it relates to the human body, its function and diseases
- Anatomy of the mouth and jaw
- Diseases of the mouth
- Basic principles of oral diagnosis and treatment, with practice on
  models of the mouth and teeth

Toward the end of the second year, students may begin to treat patients in the school's clinic, depending on the individual curriculum.

What Is Accreditation?

Early in their history, dental schools, like their medical counterparts, decided what they would teach, how long the course to become a dentist would be and what qualifications faculty had to have. Some of these schools graduated competent (for their day) practitioners; many did not.

Accreditation is one process the profession established to bring order to the chaos. It means that a school's faculty, facilities and courses meet an agreed-upon set of minimal standards. Used in conjunction with national examinations and licensing laws, accreditation helps assure that all dentists have been taught the fundamentals and have practiced their skills under supervision, achieving at least a minimal level of competence.

Programs that educate general dentists, specialists, hygienists, assistants and laboratory technicians can apply for accreditation by the Commission on Dental Accreditation of the American Dental Association. The commission is a private organization that reviews a program's curriculum and activities against a set of standards developed by the commission. Most of its 20 members are appointed by the American Dental Association, American Association of Dental Examiners, American Association of Dental Schools, dental specialty organizations, the American Dental Assistants Association, the American Dental Hygienists' Association and the National Association of Dental Laboratories. The rest of the board consists of a dental student and two members from the general public.

The review process includes a site visit by a team of consultants trained to evaluate according to commission standards and knowledgeable in the area being evaluated. These comprehensive visits are made before a program graduates its first students and every seven years thereafter (five years for oral and maxillofacial surgery programs). In addition, to retain accredita-

continued

tion, programs must submit annual reports to the commission, which can call for a special site visit if significant changes have been made in a program.

The on-site visits include interviews with school administrators, faculty and students; review of patient records, curriculum descriptions and other documents; observations of patient care; and review of a self-study report that the program completed before the visit. At the end of the visit, the group gives an oral summary of its findings to the program's administrators, followed by a written draft report. The report notes the program's strengths and weaknesses and suggests ways to improve. After rebuttal by the school, the commission issues its decision: approval, for programs that meet or exceed the standards; conditional approval, indicating that a program has specific weaknesses in one or more basic areas, which can be corrected within two years; and provisional approval, for programs with a number of significant weaknesses. In such cases, the program has a year to demonstrate measurable improvement or risk loss of accreditation. The commission has been criticized for not immediately closing these programs but asserts that its goal is to improve the quality of education, not close programs.

Theoretically, applying for accreditation is a voluntary process. But since state licensing laws require that dentists and hygienists graduate from accredited schools, programs to train them have little choice.

The accreditation process assures that all programs are reviewed by an independent body and measured against a single set of standards. However, there is still considerable variation in dental education. One study found that of 22 dentists who had graduated from American dental schools between 1980 and 1990, one had never treated a child, and half of them had no experience administering sedatives, surgically removing a tooth or performing hospital-based emergency room or operating room dental care.

The third and fourth years focus on applying the basic knowledge to actual patients. Students learn fundamental techniques of the following:

- Oral surgery
- Orthodontics
- Pediatric dentistry
- Endodontics
- Restorative dentistry (fillings and artificial crowns)
- Practice management

Most important, they work directly with patients in the school's clinic, within an affiliated hospital and in community clinics operated by or affiliated with the dental school.

Dentists who have graduated from dental schools outside the United States and who want to practice in this country complete the third and fourth years of American dental school before becoming eligible to take the licensing examination.

During their schooling, dentists must take and pass two written National Dental Examinations, also known as National Boards. Part I, taken at the end of the second year of dental school, covers anatomy, biology, chemistry and other basic academic topics. Part II is given during the fourth year and covers topics related to dental patient care, such as how to diagnose and treat specific conditions based on case examples. Successfully passing these tests is one requirement for future state licensing.

On graduation, the students receive either the Doctor of Dental Medicine (D.M.D.) or Doctor of Dental Surgery (D.D.S.) degree, depending on the school they attend. About one-third grant the D.M.D. degree. According to the American Dental Association, D.M.D. and D.D.S. degrees are equivalent because all students are graduated from similar programs with identical accreditation requirements. In 1993, the *Journal of the American Dental Association* published an editorial advocating the creation of one degree. Florida already allows dentists licensed there to use either degree designation. The bottom line is that neither degree confers more dental training or better care.

THE LICENSING PROCESS. All states require dentists to be licensed in order to practice. Thirty-nine states participate in one of four regional examinations, administered by regional examining boards; the other states have individual licensing boards that give their own licensing examination. Most states with regional examinations also require dentists to take a written examination on individual state laws related to dental and medical practice.

Licensing examinations, also known as state board examinations, have two parts. Content varies by state or region, but the written portion tends to focus on laws, medical emergency procedures, diagnosis and treatment. The second part requires applicants to demonstrate their knowledge and skill by carrying out a specified procedure on an actual patient (supplied by the applicant).

To practice, then, a dentist must:
- Pay a fee
- Pass the state/regional licensing examinations
- Pass the National Board examinations
- Produce a dental school transcript and diploma

In some states, he must also:
- Show evidence of "good moral character"
- Present a current certificate in cardiopulmonary resuscitation (CPR)
- Show evidence of malpractice insurance coverage

Having done all this, the dentist may now practice dentistry—in the state issuing the license. If he wants to practice in another state, he may have to repeat the process. According to the American Student Dental Association, 12 states do not recognize a license from another state—Alabama, Arizona, California, Florida, Georgia, Hawaii, Mississippi, New Mexico, North Carolina, Oregon, Tennessee and Texas. (There's no way to know whether this restriction is to protect "home-grown" dentists from competition, a state's citizens from less-prepared dentists or the state from "interference" from outside forces.)

Once licensed, dentists have several options. They can become employees of other dentists, clinics or HMOs. They can join the U.S. Public Health Service Corps, which is a federal government program that, among other things, provides medical and dental care to migrant workers, federal prisoners, Native Americans and other groups with little or no access to private health care. Another option, chosen by about

20 percent of graduates today, is to go into practice alone or with a partner. Finally, about 36 percent of graduates will choose to continue their education, either in a specialty (11 percent) or with additional training in general dentistry (25 percent).

Continuing Their Education

While experience counts, you also want a dentist who keeps up with new procedures, research on causes of dental disease, and the newer studies on the effectiveness of traditional procedures. And this is where continuing education comes in.

Once in practice, a dentist may never again have anyone evaluate his skills or question his knowledge of the latest dental information—except an alert patient. Health law attorney Karen Guarino, R.N., J.D., in an article in the *Journal of Dental Education,* points out that the prevalence of one-dentist offices provides little day-to-day contact with colleagues. Peer oversight is also absent because relatively few dentists practice in hospitals, where peer review and quality assurance are systematic. Dental managed care programs are not yet widespread enough and so do not provide another level of oversight.

Once a dentist passes a state's licensing examination, he is not subject to further examination unless he applies for a license in another state. Ten states require no continuing education for license renewal. And of those that do require evidence of continuing education, most only ask that dentists acknowledge they've taken the required number of hours when they submit their license renewal form, subject to a random audit. The number of hours varies considerably from state to state, ranging from 12 to 25 per year.

So in your search for the right dentist for you, be sure to ask potential dentists about their efforts to stay current.

continued

STATES REQUIRING CONTINUING EDUCATION
FOR LICENSE RENEWAL

	DENTIST	HYGIENIST	ASSISTANT
Alabama	X	X	
Alaska	X	X	
Arizona			
Arkansas	X	X	
California	X	X	X
Colorado			
Connecticut		X	
Delaware	X	X	
District of Columbia	X	X	
Florida	X	X	
Georgia	X	X	
Hawaii			
Idaho	X	X	
Illinois	X	X	
Indiana	X	X	
Iowa	X	X	
Kansas	X	X	
Kentucky	X	X	
Louisiana	X	X	
Maine	X	X	
Maryland	X	X	
Massachusetts	X	X	
Michigan	X	X	X
Minnesota	X	X	X
Mississippi	X	X	

continued

STATES REQUIRING CONTINUING EDUCATION
FOR LICENSE RENEWAL *continued*

	DENTIST	HYGIENIST	ASSISTANT
Missouri	X	X	
Montana	X	X	
Nebraska	X	X	
Nevada	X	X	
New Hampshire	X	X	X
New Jersey	X	X	
New Mexico	X	X	
New York	X	X	
North Carolina	X	X	
North Dakota	X	X	X
Ohio	X	X	
Oklahoma	X	X	
Oregon	X	X	
Pennsylvania			
Rhode Island	X	X	
South Carolina	X	X	
South Dakota	X	X	X
Tennessee	X	X	X
Texas	X	X	
Utah			
Vermont		X	
Virginia	X	X	
Washington		X	
West Virginia	X	X	
Wisconsin			
Wyoming			

DENTAL POSTGRADUATE EDUCATION. As we described earlier, dentistry recognizes eight specialties. The American Dental Association Code of Ethics requires that a dentist complete an ADA-accredited specialty training program and practice that specialty exclusively in order to identify himself as a specialist. The length of the training varies by specialty: public health dentistry, endodontics, pediatric dentistry and periodontics are two-year programs; oral pathology and orthodontics are three years long; and specialists in oral and maxillofacial surgery and prosthodontics must complete four years of postgraduate education. Most programs are hospital-based and include dental care of hospitalized patients and clients in outpatient dental clinics, and time in laboratories and operating rooms, depending on the specialty. Instruction, which includes both lectures and patient care, goes beyond the introduction provided during undergraduate dental training and focuses on developing skills and knowledge in depth of topics within the specialty.

Postgraduate training for general dentists became formalized in 1972. The yearlong programs provide training in areas not fully covered during the busy undergraduate years, including use of sedatives, emergency medicine and anesthesiology. In addition, many of the programs emphasize the care of medically compromised patients such as those with heart disease, AIDS and other infectious diseases, diabetes and cancer, as well as physically and mentally handicapped patients. It is not considered another specialty, the way family practice has become in medicine.

The choice of completing a postgraduate year in general dentistry is entirely voluntary and is currently made by about 25 percent of dental school graduates. Individuals who enter the postgraduate general dentistry programs are generally those who ranked high in their undergraduate programs, according to Lawrence Meskin, D.D.S., editor of the *Journal of the American Dental Association*. Studies have found that practicing dentists who completed a postgraduate general dentistry program tended to spend more time caring for patients in hospitals and nursing homes, referred patients to specialists less often and prescribed fewer pain relievers and antibiotics than did general dentists who had entered practice right after dental school. However, the researchers did not evaluate the overall quality of care patients received by either type of dentist.

Relatively few general dentists choose to formally continue their education, so you are unlikely to find such a practitioner without a diligent search. A typical profile of a dentist who has completed a postgraduate general dentistry program might read something like this: He is most likely to have graduated from dental school since the early 1980s, when the size of many postgraduate programs significantly increased. He also probably has admitting privileges to a local hospital and teaches at a nearby dental school (both are potential referral resources).

WHAT ABOUT BOARD CERTIFICATION? Certification plays a much less significant role for dental specialists than for most medical specialists. Once a dentist has successfully completed his specialty education, he can practice that specialty throughout his career without applying for board certification. Physicians, on the other hand, are pressured by hospitals and powerful managed care plans to become certified. Dental specialists in oral surgery and others who treat patients in hospitals may have to seek certification as a requirement for hospital admitting privileges. Furthermore, as managed care becomes more common in dentistry, the managed care companies will be pressuring specialists who want to be part of the company's network to become certified.

To be eligible to take the certification examination, specialists must have not only the specialty education described above but also work experience: Oral surgeons and orthodontists must practice at least one year after completing their specialty education; endodontists, oral pathologists and pediatric dentists, two years; periodontists, three years; and public health dentists, four years. All applicants complete a written test. Oral pathologists must also demonstrate their skills at examining various tissues. All other specialties add oral questioning and a presentation of a patient's case history. Certification for pediatric dentistry includes an examination of an actual patient.

Once certified, only specialists in oral and maxillofacial surgery, pediatric dentistry and prosthodontics must be recertified by examination at regular intervals. Otherwise, all that is required is to fill out a reregistration form and pay a fee each year. No specialty board has ever revoked a certificate.

Now let's look at the other people we might expect to encounter in the dental setting.

The Other Players on Your Dental Health Team

The typical dental office has three staff members in addition to the dentist to help care for you: a business office assistant, a dental (chairside) assistant and a hygienist. In the dental profession, these are commonly called auxiliaries. A large office with several dentists may have more than one chairside assistant or hygienist, as well as an office manager who oversees the day-to-day running of the business side of the office; a care coordinator who monitors patient scheduling and answers general patient questions about care; a bookkeeper/records technician who handles billings and dental records; and possibly a laboratory technician who prepares bridges, dentures and other replacement teeth.

OFFICE ASSISTANTS. Office assistants typically answer the telephone, make appointments, handle billings and payments and help run the office. They may have completed a short commercial course in medical office management or have received on-the-job training. While their responsibilities don't relate directly to the care you receive, they are nevertheless an important element in your overall comfort and confidence in the practice. A competent office assistant enables the dentist and hygienist to concentrate on your care; she can be depended on to remind you about appointments, to send recall notices and to assist you in arranging for installment payments.

DENTAL ASSISTANTS. Dental assistants work chairside with the dentist in providing care. In testimony before the American Association of Dental Schools in late 1995, then-president-elect Jennifer Blake of the American Dental Assistant Association noted, "Dental assistants are the only dental health care professionals delivering intraoral services to the public who are not mandated to satisfy certain educational requirements or to be credentialed." Only five states—Arkansas, California, Michigan, Minnesota and New Jersey—require that they register with the state in order to practice.

In fact, more than half are trained on the job by the dentists who employ them. Others will have completed a yearlong course in a commercial business school, junior or community college, and even a few dental schools. About half the programs are accredited by the Com-

Dental Supervision

Your state's dental practice act specifies the duties that a dental hygienist or assistant can carry out under any of four levels of supervision by a dentist.

Direct supervision means that the dentist:
- Personally authorized the procedure
- Is in the office while the task is being carried out
- Personally reviews the work before the patient leaves the office

Indirect supervision indicates that the dentist:
- Has authorized the procedure based on his diagnosis
- Is in the office while the task is being carried out

General supervision means that the dentist:
- Has authorized the procedure based on his diagnosis
- Does not have to be present while the delegated task is being performed
- Remains legally responsible for the work and is expected to delegate only to qualified staff

Personal supervision refers to circumstances under which the hygienist/assistant assists the dentist as he carries out a procedure.

mission on Dental Accreditation of the American Dental Association, the same group that accredits dental schools. The curriculum of these accredited programs includes psychology, anatomy, nutrition, dental x-ray techniques, emergency procedures, ethics, office management and practice in assisting with patients.

A voluntary certification program requires current CPR certification and course work in radiation health and safety, infection control and general chairside topics such as applying topical (noninjected) anesthetics and removing excess cement after a crown has been installed. The independent nonprofit Dental Assisting National Board conducts the certify-

State Dental Practice Acts

State dental practice acts are the set of laws governing the practice of dentistry in your state. They regulate the licensing and responsibilities of dentists and of dental auxiliaries, including hygienists, assistants and laboratory technicians. The act authorizes an administrative board, called the state board of dental examiners in most states. There are considerable variations among states in what is legally permitted or required—for example, one in three states has no education or examination requirements for a dental professional to be able to take x-rays. Consequently, you cannot assume that the laws are protecting your best interests. If you have any questions about licensing or what tasks can legally be performed, call your state board of dental examiners.

ing examinations and awards certification in four areas: Certified Dental Assistant, Certified Orthodontic Assistant, Certified Oral and Maxillofacial Surgery Assistant and Certified Dental Practice Management Assistant. Certified assistants must also complete 12 hours of approved continuing education each year to maintain their credentials. Of the estimated 200,000 dental assistants in the United States, about 29,000 have been certified by the board.

Certified or not, dental assistants work directly under the supervision of dentists and hygienists. Assistants are usually responsible for sterilizing instruments and following infection control protocols, as we describe in the next chapter. They also prepare the operatory (chairside area) for each patient, replacing disposable headrest covers, putting instruments on the dentist's work tray, disinfecting work surfaces and performing any other related tasks. Depending on state law and the dentist's delegation preferences, assistants may carry out various hands-on tasks such as mixing amalgam materials, applying topical fluoride and removing a temporary tooth.

DENTAL HYGIENISTS. Most commonly, the functions performed by dental hygienists include teeth cleaning, nutrition counseling and patient education about home oral care. In recent years, states have revised their practice laws to allow hygienists a broader scope of practice. For example, 14 states now allow them to administer nitrous oxide anesthetic if the dentist is in the office. And all states permit them to carry out sealant application and root planing—some states require a dentist to be present during such procedures, and others do not.

What Your Hygienist Can Do

In general, the functions that hygienists can perform are those that are reversible. For example, they cannot drill a tooth to prepare it for an amalgam restoration (silver filling), but they can polish the amalgam once the dentist has put it into place. This list shows the functions that can be performed in at least one state. Those with an asterisk can be performed by hygienists in all states.

Perform prophylaxis*	Place sutures
Take x-rays*	Remove sutures
Administer local anesthesia	Apply cavity liners and bases
Administer topical anesthesia	Place temporary restorations
Apply fluoride*	Remove temporary restorations
Apply pit/fissure sealants*	Place amalgam restorations
Perform root planing*	Carve amalgam restorations
Perform soft tissue curettage	Finish amalgam restorations
Administer nitrous oxide	Polish amalgam restorations*
Take study cast impressions	Place and finish composite
Place periodontal dressing	resin silicate restorations

Source: American Dental Hygienists' Association.

At a minimum, hygienists are required to complete a two-year associate degree program at a college-level hygiene program accredited by the Commission on Dental Accreditation of the American Dental Association. Bachelor's and master's degree programs are also available, primarily to prepare hygienists to teach, conduct research and administer hygiene programs in large government and private dental clinics. The associate-degree curriculum includes both basic dental science courses and clinical experience treating patients under supervision. Graduates must pass a national board examination, earning the registered dental hygienist designation.

To receive a state license to practice, they must also pass a state or regional licensing examination that includes a written test and a clinical test on actual patients. Forty-two states, the District of Columbia and Puerto Rico also require hygienists to take accredited continuing education courses in order to earn license renewal.

The first dental hygienist was trained by a Connecticut dentist in 1906, primarily to perform cleanings and other preventive treatments. In the 1960s, the first experiments to significantly expand the duties of dental hygienists and assistants began. Most changes in state laws to allow additional responsibilities, however, have taken place within the past decade. Currently, 29 functions are legal in at least some states. Call your state board of dental examiners (called a board of dentistry in some states) for details about your state laws.

Be aware, however, that studies have found that dentists often delegate functions without regard for state law. For example, nearly a quarter of dentists surveyed in Grand Rapids, Michigan, reported that they delegated pumice polishing (using a mild abrasive paste to remove teeth stains) to their dental assistants, despite the fact that Michigan law did not allow assistants to carry out the procedure. More important, perhaps, is the finding from studies in Kentucky and Washington State that the quality of the expanded functions performed by assistants and hygienists was closely related to the quality of the dentist's work. So, while you want to ask about the training of assistants and hygienists who will help care for you, your primary concern must be for the supervising dentist, whose competency affects not only the care he provides but that of other team members as well.

Hygienists Go It Alone

In the late 1980s, California dental hygienists started an experiment to evaluate the benefits and risks of independent practices by hygienists. Thirty-four registered hygienists completed 118 hours of additional instruction and a 300-hour practicum in which they carried out expanded duties and responsibilities related to running a practice while employed by a dentist. Ten pilot practices were eventually set up across the state, some serving nursing home and other institutional clients, one offering services in clients' homes, and the others in office settings. Among the services they provided were cleaning and preliminary examination, x-rays, topical fluoride applications and patient education—all without direct supervision by a dentist. Practices were evaluated by a team of dentists/evaluators before opening and twice annually to help protect patient health and safety.

These start-up hygienist practices had lower fees than did the dentists in the area for similar services. The hygienists were also more willing to take on Medicaid patients than the dentists.

Several attempts were made during the early 1990s to pass legislation to enable these pilot practices and others to be established permanently in California. To date, these efforts have failed by slim margins. The pilot project was in its final stage by early 1997.

Several states, including Colorado and Washington State, have passed or are considering laws to allow independent practice by hygienists. These professionals cannot supply all of your dental care; a dentist must still carry out procedures under local or general anesthesia. However, an independent hygienist may be a viable alternative for patients who want to maintain basic preventive measures between major dental examinations, who live in underserved areas or who have circumstances that make a visit to a dentist's office difficult (such as those who are homebound).

As we've said, dental care is a highly personal service, and finding the "right" dentist for you is an essential first step to getting quality care. But where you get that care matters as well. In the next chapter, we help you evaluate the safety, appropriateness and convenience of your dentist's office and other dental settings.

Where You Go for Dental Care

ith the exception of major surgery—to correct a cleft palate or repair facial bones broken in an accident, for example—the choice of where you get dental care has less to do with the type of procedure and more with specific conditions you might have. Almost every dental procedure (except major surgery) *can be* and *is* performed in any of the three main types of settings—the office, the ambulatory care (outpatient, same-day surgery) center and the hospital. Before we consider issues involved in evaluating each setting, let's look at some of the conditions that might affect where you get your dental care.

- *Level of anxiety.* People who have intense dental anxiety may be referred to ambulatory care centers or hospitals to have procedures done under sedation or general anesthesia. In addition, a few hospitals, such as the Mount Sinai Medical Center in New York, have created dental phobia clinics to provide both dental care and counseling to decrease the fear.

- *Disability.* Physically challenged patients, especially those with cerebral palsy or other diseases that affect muscle control, and mentally challenged patients need careful monitoring and perhaps sedation during dental care; even basic procedures such as restorations (fillings) are likely to be performed in an ambulatory care center if available or in a hospital.

■ **Medical condition.** In medical parlance, people with preexisting medical conditions that could affect the outcome of a procedure are referred to as medically compromised. These include individuals with chronic illnesses such as heart disease, lung disease, high blood pressure and cirrhosis and other liver diseases, as well as people with active infectious diseases such as tuberculosis or anyone undergoing radiation therapy for cancer. Such patients often require laboratory tests and evaluations and close monitoring by their physicians when dental procedures must be done. Often their care is provided in hospitals.

■ **Dental condition.** People who need extensive dental care in one visit will likely be referred to an ambulatory center or hospital. Among these circumstances are a toddler with nursing bottle cavities (multiple cavities in front teeth from sucking on a bottle during sleep); a patient with facial injuries needing a team of specialists to surgically correct them; or an adult who needs several root canal procedures (to remove the root and eliminate infection) done in one sitting because he or she cannot schedule several routine office appointments to carry out the therapy.

If, on the other hand, you're healthy, you'll probably receive your care in the office if you need any of the following procedures:

■ Restorations, both fillings and artificial crowns
■ Extractions—i.e., removal of one or more teeth
■ Root canal therapy that removes the root, cleans the canal and prepares the remaining structure for a crown
■ Orthodontic therapy to straighten teeth
■ Periodontic therapy to eliminate gum disease and repair damage to gum and bone from bacteria
■ Denture preparation and fittings

Just what can you expect when you get care in a dental office? And what potential dental hazards should you know about?

YOUR DENTIST'S OFFICE

Dentistry remains overwhelmingly office-based. You're likely to find these offices in medical/professional buildings, health maintenance organization clinics, shopping centers and malls and, of course, in self-contained, stand-alone offices. Whether the office is in a converted house or an ultramodern building, its general layout is likely to be similar. During your get-acquainted visit, take a moment to familiarize yourself with the surroundings. This will help you put into context the various aspects of office safety we discuss later in this chapter.

The Layout

As you look around, you will probably find the following areas:

- Patient waiting area
- One or more patient treatment areas, known as operatories
- Front office/medical records/billing room
- Laboratory for sterilization of instruments and adjustment of dental appliances such as dentures and partial bridges
- X-ray development area or darkroom
- Dentist's private office/consultation room

The greater the number of dentists in the practice, the greater the likelihood that you will find all these rooms.

Within a typical operatory may be various cabinets and drawers for supplies, an x-ray machine, an electrically controlled reclining chair for the patient and wheeled chair(s) for the dentist/hygienist, two sinks, an adjustable overhead light, a saliva ejector (a small suction pump and hose with a disposable tip), an air compressor and hoses that power the handpiece with its detachable heads and tips, and the instrument tray. You may also see an ultrasonic cleaning machine for removing tartar and plaque and a video camera and monitor for viewing your teeth and gums.

All rooms should be clean and uncluttered. Patient areas should be brightly lit. Furnishings and equipment should not be worn or broken. Look for an environment that calms you and contributes to your physical and emotional comfort. The availability of patient education brochures, videos and/or health and fitness magazines is one indicator of a dentist who encourages patient participation and preventive dentistry.

Even the best-looking office, however, can harbor health hazards for you if you are an unwary dental consumer. Slipshod office procedures and inadequate or defective equipment can spell disaster in an emergency or expose you to unnecessary risks of infection or excessive x-rays. So take time during your get-acquainted visit to evaluate the office's safety, based on the following information.

Budget Alternatives

If the cost of dental care in a private office has kept you from seeking care, you may want to investigate the availability of any of several lower-cost alternatives.

Government Clinics

The federal government funds more than 550 clinics called community health centers in designated medically underserved areas. These clinics are required to provide preventive dental care, especially for children and adolescents, who comprise about one-third of patients seen in these clinics. About half of the facilities also provide primary care services such as fillings.

Active duty military personnel receive comprehensive dental care through the Department of Defense medical system. While active duty personnel have first priority, their families and retirees can also receive dental care through this system, including emergencies, routine preventive care and restorative procedures such as fillings and crowns.

The Veterans Administration provides dental services for both service-connected and nonservice-connected visits to those patients who qualify for VA benefits by virtue of service-related disability.

Despite significant funding cuts, about 140 dental clinics, sponsored by city or county governments, are available. You may also find that major hospitals that operate outpatient medical clinics for Medicaid recipients and other people with low incomes may also provide at least some dental services. In all cases, services and administrative policies vary significantly from program to program, as do fees. Many use a sliding fee scale or copayment system, with fees based on your ability to pay. Be prepared to substantiate your financial circumstances and other qualifications, such as union membership or former military service.   *continued*

In 1986, researchers at Ohio State University analyzed local dental clinics in 31 states. Almost all of the 144 clinics provided preventive care such as cleanings, basic restorative care such as fillings, and emergency care. Almost none provided orthodontic care. This survey also found that over a quarter of the clinics had no program in place to evaluate the quality of care, less than half required dentists to wear gloves with all patients, and only a quarter required staff to be vaccinated against hepatitis B. If you seek care in any low-cost facility, do not accept substandard care. Ask the questions we've outlined; insist that basic infection control procedures be carried out.

Dental School Clinics

Another low-cost alternative is available to those who live near a dental school. In order to provide patient-care experience for their students, these schools operate clinics in which third- and fourth-year students carry out procedures under the direct supervision of faculty. As a general rule, these clinics do not emphasize prevention; the students are there primarily to learn to restore teeth, perform root canals and practice applying other "hands-on" techniques.

The Many Sides of Safety

EMERGENCY PREPAREDNESS. Two surveys of more than 4,300 dentists, reported in 1992, found that during a 10-year period, each dentist experienced an average of seven medical emergencies resulting from dental care. The most common emergency, fainting—which can be caused by anxiety, among other factors—accounted for half the emergencies reported. Depending upon the individual circumstances, fainting sometimes carries the risks associated with a drop in blood pressure, breathing difficulties and central nervous system disruption. A person with diabetes who doesn't eat before a visit may experience dangerous blood-sugar levels. An allergy to anesthesia may cause serious breathing problems.

While these conditions are serious, they are reversible if prompt and appropriate medical care is provided. Unfortunately, a general dentist's education "provides little preparation for management of life-and-death situations," comment Robert M. Peskin, D.D.S., and Louis I. Siegelman, D.D.S., in a 1995 article in *Dental Clinics of North America*. Yet responsibility for emergency management rests solely with the dentist, because government oversight of the dental office is minimal or nonexistent. Inspections may come only as a result of consumer complaints or focus on other aspects of safety such as infection control or x-ray equipment.

Your get-acquainted visit gives you a chance to ask some basic questions about your dentist's ability to handle emergencies:

1. What training in medical emergency management have you had?

Six of 10 dental schools do not have a separate course in emergency training, but instead incorporate the topic into other courses. As a result, general dentists may have 10 or fewer hours of emergency training during dental school. And they probably had no experience in applying that training because only 22 percent of dental schools conduct emergency drills. Students are required to be certified in cardiopulmonary resuscitation (CPR) at the start of their schooling, but one in eight dental schools has no program to maintain certification throughout the four-year program. Furthermore, after graduation dentists may allow their certification to lapse if they live in a state that doesn't require CPR certification for licensing. Dentists who complete postgraduate work to specialize in pediatric dentistry, oral surgery or dental anesthesiology have additional courses in medical emergency management during their residency, and must be certified in advanced cardiac life support (ACLS). Training in ACLS includes the proper use of cardiac monitors, oxygen administration and intravenous medications to stimulate the heart in emergencies.

Dental hygienists must also be certified in CPR during their training. They receive between one and 64 hours of medical emergency training, depending on the school, with two-thirds of schools incorporating the subject into other courses. In 45 percent of hygienist schools, students test their preparedness with emergency drills.

Most states test knowledge of emergency procedures on the written portion of their licensing examination for dentists and hygienists.

CPR Requirements for Dentists—
Where Does Your State Stand?

The following states require that dentists be trained in cardio-pulmonary resuscitation (CPR) either at initial licensing or at renewal, or both. Contact your state board of dental examiners for details.

Alabama	Kentucky	Oklahoma
Alaska	Louisiana	Oregon
Arizona	Maryland	South Carolina
California	Mississippi	South Dakota
Colorado	Missouri	Tennessee
Delaware	Montana	Texas
Florida	Nevada	Utah
Georgia	New Mexico	Vermont
Idaho	North Carolina	Wisconsin
Indiana	North Dakota	

Source: American Dental Association, American Student Dental Association.

2. What plans do you have in place for dealing with emergencies?

Peskin and Siegelman provide a checklist for dentists to prepare themselves and their staffs for emergencies. It can also serve as a guideline as you visit prospective offices and talk with dentists and their staffs.

Find out the following:

- Are all staff members currently certified in CPR?
- Do all staff members have assigned tasks in case of emergency?
- Have contingency plans been made to cover all emergency tasks in the event a staff member is absent?

- Are periodic unannounced mock emergency drills carried out?
- Are appropriate emergency telephone numbers posted prominently next to all telephones?
- Is the oxygen tank checked regularly? And is other emergency equipment on hand, in good working order, and located where the emergency plan indicates?
- Are all emergency medications checked weekly and replaced when used or expired?
- Has a specific staff member been assigned to complete this checklist regularly?

Adapted from Robert M. Peskin and Louis I. Siegelman, "Emergency Cardiac Care: Moral, Legal and Ethical Considerations," *Dental Clinics of North America* 39, no. 3 (1995): pp. 677-688.

INFECTION CONTROL. The need for patients to be vigilant for potential gaps in an office's infection control procedures is unfortunately very real. Any virus or bacteria carried by blood, such as the hepatitis virus, or by saliva, such as the tuberculosis virus, can potentially be transmitted in a dental office. At least nine dental workers infected 147 patients with hepatitis B virus between 1970 and 1987, and one dentist infected six patients with the human immunodeficiency virus in the early 1990s. Because the source of an infection can be very difficult to trace in isolated cases, the actual number of patients infected by the various viruses and bacteria commonly found in modern dental offices is likely to be much greater.

Transmission of infectious diseases to dental patients can happen via three routes. First, the dentist (or hygienist) who is infected passes the illness on to the patient through blood from a cut on the dentist's ungloved hand. Second, equipment or instruments contaminated by one patient and not properly sterilized can pass illness on to another patient. Third, airborne contaminants in saliva droplets from the infected dentist's unmasked face can transmit disease during therapy.

In 1991, the Occupational Safety and Health Administration (OSHA) issued standards to protect employees of dental offices from infection. Many of the standards, enacted into federal law, simultaneously protect patients. For example, workers are required to wear gloves and masks.

The law also allows OSHA to inspect dental offices and issue fines for offenders. However, inspections are not mandatory for all offices, but instead come as the result of employee complaints. Again, the emphasis of these inspections is on employee protection, not patient safety.

Guidelines for effective infection control have also been issued by the Centers for Disease Control and Prevention and the American Dental Association. However, these do not carry the force of law or impose penalties on dentists who do not follow the guidelines.

At the state level, the examination that dentists take for initial licensing, described in chapter 1, includes questions about proper infection control procedures. This, of course, tests knowledge, not actual practice. To find out if your state goes further and inspects dental offices for infection control measures, call your state board of dental examiners. In most cases, you'll find that no one regularly monitors a dentist's compliance with infection control standards—no one except you, the alert consumer.

Consistency is essential in applying infection control procedures. This concept, initiated by the Centers for Disease Control and Prevention, is known as universal precautions. It means that procedures are carried out as if all patients' blood and saliva carry infectious agents. In other words, the same precautions are used for all patients. The dentist who thinks that she needs to practice infection control only with patients she believes are high risk is endangering herself, her staff and her other patients. Yet studies repeatedly show that some dentists and their staffs apply the guidelines only when it is convenient or they believe a risk exists.

During a brief get-acquainted visit, of course, you cannot observe consistent behavior over time. You also cannot observe how well some of the procedures are actually carried out because they take place before the office opens. Nevertheless, there are questions you can ask and some activities you can observe. Once you have selected a dentist, you will have to remain vigilant before and during dental procedures. See chapter 3 for additional information about specific infection control procedures, including those that involve dental equipment.

Here, let's look at what infection control procedures are supposed to accomplish. As we've noted, infection can be transmitted via direct contact with blood or other body fluids, indirect contact with contaminated instruments or equipment or contact with airborne contaminants such as droplets from a cough. Three things are needed in order for infection to occur: (a) a susceptible host (patient or dental worker), (b) virus or bacteria at levels high enough to cause disease and (c) a way for the virus to enter the body (mouth or nose). Infection control procedures are designed to eliminate one or more of these elements, thus preventing a complete cycle and infection. To learn more about how your dentist protects you, ask the following:

1. Do you have a written infection control plan? Who is responsible for carrying it out? What training does she have?

Every dental office should have a written infection control plan in place that outlines the procedures to be followed, when they are to be used and who is responsible for carrying them out. Ask to see the plan in any office you visit.

Having a written plan doesn't ensure that it is followed, of course. A study of disinfection of clean water units designed to provide water, independent of the local water supply, to the dental handpiece and water syringe found that only one dentist in five was following the manufacturer's written instructions for disinfection. Your own questions and observations can help verify in at least some instances that infection control procedures are being carried out as written.

You can't see them, of course, but bacteria and viruses cling to instruments and equipment. Any effective infection control process must include these items. The Centers for Disease Control and Prevention recommend the following:

- All instruments that penetrate gums or bone or come into direct contact with mouth tissues should be cleaned, preferably by an ultrasonic device, and then sterilized with heat between each use.

- Instruments that are not being used immediately after sterilization should be packaged for storage.

- Items such as the handle of the examining light or x-ray unit heads should be covered with plastic, aluminum foil or other barriers that are changed after use with each patient.

▪ After each patient and at the end of the day, countertops and other surfaces in patient care areas should be wiped with disposable towels and disinfected with a solution of bleach and water or a germicide labeled as a "hospital disinfectant" and "tuberculocidal," in the latter case meaning that it is effective against the tuberculosis bacterium.

▪ After each patient, water lines to the high-speed handpiece and water syringe should be run 20 to 30 seconds to flush water and air into a sink or container. They should also be flushed for two to three minutes at the beginning of each day.

▪ Whenever possible, disposable instruments should be used—for example, the tip of saliva ejectors or cleaning brushes—and replaced after each patient.

An assistant or hygienist usually carries out most or all of these tasks, so you may want to ask her, in addition to the dentist, about how they are handled in the office. Some dentists recognize that infection protection is important to patients and have prepared brochures or letters describing their efforts. Ask if one is available.

Both the staff and the equipment need to be scrutinized. For example, anyone working in your mouth should wash her hands before starting; she should wear latex or vinyl gloves, eyeglasses and a surgical mask (or a plastic face shield that covers eyes, nose and mouth). She should also wear protective clothing such as a laboratory coat, uniform or disposable gown, which is changed daily or when it becomes visibly soiled. A 1992 study of Chicago dentists found that while 90 percent wore gloves and 79 percent wore protective clothing, only about 62 percent wore either a face mask or eye protection. These items are fundamental to infection control today; do not even consider a dentist who does not follow these basic procedures.

2. Do you take a written medical and dental history for new patients? How often do you update it?

A complete history should be taken when you first become a patient and updated at each office visit. Between 75 and 90 percent of the Chicago dentists surveyed took an initial history. However, other studies have found that as few as one in three dentists take an initial history and make regular updates.

3. Have you and your staff been vaccinated against hepatitis B? Do you have annual tuberculosis tests?

The dentist and her staff should be vaccinated against hepatitis B virus. Hepatitis B is a disease of the liver that can be transmitted by the blood of an infected person. It can become chronic and lead to cirrhosis and other liver damage. Hepatitis B infection is the most commonly acquired blood-borne infection found in dental workers. Dentists have almost twice the rate of infection as the general population, even with the availability of a vaccine, introduced in 1982. According to an American Dental Association survey, 85 percent of dentists reported receiving the vaccine by 1992. The survey found that the longer a dentist had been in practice, the less likely she was to have had the vaccine and the more likely she was to have been infected.

OSHA now requires all dental workers who come into direct contact with patients to be vaccinated against hepatitis B. The vaccine protects them from infection by the hepatitis B virus and thereby from passing it on to you and other patients.

If you live in a major metropolitan area, each dental employee should undergo annual tests for tuberculosis. This is particularly true in New York, California and Texas, where the rate of reported tuberculosis cases in the general population rose 84 percent, 54 percent and 33 percent, respectively, between 1985 and 1992.

X-RAY SAFETY. In modern dentistry, an x-ray examination is the only way that dental diseases below the gum line or inside the tooth can be diagnosed. Without x-rays, specialized dental work such as root canal therapy and orthodontics cannot be done.

But x-rays, even the low-level x-rays of dentistry, still carry risks. In 1995, Robert P. Langlais, D.D.S., M.S., and Olaf E. Langland, D.D.S., M.S., from the University of Texas Health Science Center at San Antonio, published an analysis of the current risks from dental radiation. Reviewing numerous studies, Langlais and Langland made the following assessments:

■ For every million full-mouth x-ray examinations (16 to 24 views of all teeth taken at one time) performed, less than one extra case each of leukemia, lung cancer and thyroid cancer can be expected.

- Overall, for every million full-mouth x-ray examinations performed, 2.5 extra cases of cancer of all types can be expected.

- The risk of death from dental x-rays is about one in a million, comparable with smoking one cigarette or riding your bicycle for 10 miles.

- While a theoretical risk of cataract formation exists, in practice the level of radiation exposure to the eye is so low that, according to Langlais and Langland, "the risk of producing damage is remote."

Two University of California at Los Angeles professors, Susan Preston-Martin, Ph.D., and Stuart C. White, D.D.S., Ph.D., have closely examined the relationship of brain and salivary gland tumors to dental radiation. They conclude that of the eight cases of parotid gland (the largest salivary gland) cancer per million people in Los Angeles, one is caused by dental radiography. They also found that children diagnosed with brain tumors at the age of 15 to 24 years were two-and-one-half times as likely to have had five or more sets of full-mouth x-ray examinations as were young children with similar tumors.

Over the years, efforts have been made to reduce both the frequency and the radiation level of x-rays. In 1988, for example, the U.S. Food and Drug Administration issued guidelines to help dentists reduce the number of x-ray examinations performed. Those guidelines were approved by the American Dental Association and other dental organizations. If you are an adult with normal teeth and gums and no more than an occasional cavity, you can reduce your exposure by 40 percent by visiting a dentist who follows these guidelines:

- At your initial visit, bitewing views of your back teeth should be taken to provide a baseline for future comparisons as well as to identify any problems that need immediate attention. These x-rays show the crown and part of the root of two or three pairs of opposing teeth, especially the large molars at the side and back of the mouth. Bitewings may also be needed for specific circumstances, such as assisting the dentist in carrying out a root canal procedure. If you are changing dentists and have a full set in your previous medical record, ask to have it transferred to the new dentist. Bitewings should be taken every 18 to 36 months.

- Periapical x-rays show both the visible crown of the tooth and its entire root. These views are no longer recommended routinely for a healthy person's initial office visit. Periapical views should be taken only after a comprehensive examination identifies the presence of certain conditions such as unusual tooth color, pain, unexplained tooth sensitivity to temperature or pressure, or a history of periodontal disease.

Careful questioning during your get-acquainted visit will help you further reduce your risk from dental x-rays. Among the questions to ask are:

1. Who takes patient x-rays? What training and/or experience does she have? Is she certified/licensed to do so?

Equally important to the frequency of the x-ray examination is the quality of the x-ray. Modern equipment and high-speed film have made the procedure relatively simple and fast, but it is still important that the operator know what must be done to ensure accuracy, readability and patient safety. A 1996 study reported in the *Journal of the American Dental Association,* for example, found as many as 20 percent of dental x-rays were unacceptable in that they did not provide an image that was clear, undistorted or otherwise accurate enough to be useful to the dentist. Other reports have found even higher levels.

A dentist must determine the need for x-rays, but the dentist, hygienist and, in some states, assistant can take the actual x-ray. Your state dental practice act specifies who can take them and whether licensing or registration is necessary. In 1981, the federal Consumer-Patient Radiation Health and Safety Act was passed to update requirements for those who take x-rays, but many states still do not have legislation in place to carry out the federal mandate. Connecticut, for example, put into effect "An Act Concerning X-Ray Safety" in October 1993, requiring that all dental assistants who take x-rays must pass the Dental Assisting National Board's radiography examination by January 1, 1995. However, as many as 14 states still have no requirements for assistants who take radiographs.

Training for dentists and dental hygienists includes courses in radiation safety and procedures, and licensing examinations have a section on the topic. The certification program for dental assistants, described in chapter 1, includes course work and an examination on radiation safety and procedures as well.

2. What type of protective equipment do you use for patients?

During your visit, ask to see the x-ray equipment and protective devices used for patients. The equipment should have a long (about eight inches) lead-lined rectangular tube that is aligned next to your cheek, rather than a short, pointed plastic cone. The rectangular tube provides a narrow beam and exposes the least area to radiation, reducing skin exposure as much as 50 percent compared with the cone, according to several reports, including one in 1995 by Jack N. Hadley, D.D.S., assistant professor of radiology at the University of the Pacific School of Dentistry in San Francisco. Patients should wear a lead apron and collar for all x-rays to protect the thyroid gland, which is particularly susceptible to radiation, and other organs from unwarranted exposure.

3. How do you monitor the radiation dose given by the machine?

Poor maintenance and other factors can cause machines to emit more radiation than they are supposed to or is necessary. The dentist can easily monitor the dose by using an inexpensive device called a dosimeter or a radiation-monitoring-by-mail service, in which lapel badges worn by dental staff are sent on a regular basis to an off-site laboratory for calculation of exposure.

4. Do you use Ektaspeed x-ray film (also called E film)?

This is a rapid-speed, high-resolution, short-exposure film that reduces the length of time a patient is exposed to radiation compared with the previous D film. Note, however, that a survey of nearly 2,000 California dentists in 1995 found that only 21 percent were using E speed film.

While these issues of safety are important to evaluate during your get-acquainted visit and to weigh in your final choice of a dentist, they should remain issues of concern throughout your dental care. Remain alert and be willing to ask these questions about emergency preparedness, infection control and x-ray procedures anytime you suspect standards may have fallen—for example, when new staff members join the practice or the dentist seems particularly busy.

Your concern for safety carries over to other dental settings as well. Ambulatory care centers, for medical, surgical and dental care, have grown in popularity in recent decades as a result of improvements in anesthesiology, demand by managed care plans, among others, for shorter hospital stays and consumer preference. Nevertheless, if your dentist recommends that you undergo dental care at an ambulatory center, you need to evaluate it as carefully as you did the dental office and staff.

AMBULATORY CARE CENTERS

Ambulatory care centers provide care that does not require an overnight stay in a hospital. This can include medical procedures such as kidney dialysis, surgery such as cyst removal and dental procedures ranging from several restorations to implant surgery (surgery to place a metal base into the jaw to which artificial teeth can be permanently attached).

More than 28 million ambulatory surgery procedures of all kinds were performed in 1996, of which about 222,000 involved teeth, gums and tooth sockets.

Dental procedures may be performed at a general ambulatory center or one specializing in dentistry. Large hospitals (with 400 beds or more) and those affiliated with universities that train dentists are most likely to have specialized dental centers. About 1,000 U.S. hospitals have such centers. Nine of 10 hospital-owned dental centers are located within the hospital itself, with the others situated adjacent to the hospital or in a few instances at off-site, freestanding facilities.

Dental centers can also be owned and operated by dentists, individually or as part of a group, and less commonly by government agencies or nonprofit organizations.

When choosing one setting over another, quality, not convenience, must be the deciding factor.

Before you go to an outpatient center for surgical care, find out as much as possible about its facilities and staff. Visit the facility and speak with the director or other supervisory staff. In particular:

■ Find out the center's licensing and certification status. Not all states license these facilities, but if your state does, then avoid an unlicensed center. Call your state department of health to find out its responsibility and the status of the center you have chosen. Some private medical in-

When the Dentist Says Outpatient Surgery

When your dentist recommends surgery, she will indicate whether it can be done on an outpatient basis and where she would like to perform it. Among the questions you want to ask her are the following:

1. Is a nonsurgical alternative available? Why have you recommended surgery?

2. What happens if I don't have the surgery? Is there any advantage or disadvantage to waiting?

3. Will you perform the surgery? If so, how often have you done so? What complications do your patients commonly experience? Have your patients experienced any serious or permanent side effects?

4. Why do you want to do this on an outpatient basis? Does this surgery carry any additional risks when performed on an outpatient basis?

5. What percentage of patients undergoing this surgery as outpatients have been admitted to the hospital with complications necessitating an overnight stay (or longer)? What were the complications?

6. Why do you want to perform the surgery at this particular center? Could you perform it at another ambulatory center or in your office?

surers certify facilities in the areas of safety, cleanliness and preparedness for emergencies. The facility's business manager or your insurance company can tell you if it has such certification. Finally, centers can voluntarily apply for accreditation by the Joint Commission on Accreditation of Healthcare Organizations or the Accreditation Association for Ambulatory Health Care. The review process—which, by the way, the facility pays for the privilege of undergoing—evaluates quality-assurance measures, staffing and a wide range of other criteria. Unfortunately, few non-hospital-based centers have undergone the process. Most centers prominently display their certification letter, but you can also check the center your dentist has recommended by contacting either organization:

> Accreditation Association for Ambulatory Health Care
> 9933 Lawler Ave., Suite 512
> Skokie, IL 60077-3708
> 847-676-9610

> Joint Commission on Accreditation of Healthcare
> Organizations
> One Renaissance Blvd.
> Oakbrook Terrace, IL 60181
> 630-916-5600

What Is JCAHO?

The Joint Commission on Accreditation of Healthcare Organizations was founded in 1951 (as the Joint Commission on Accreditation of Hospitals) by the American College of Surgeons, the American Hospital Association, the American Medical Association, the American College of Physicians and the Canadian Medical Association (which withdrew in 1959). The American Dental Association was added in 1979.

The commission was incorporated as a private not-for-profit organization with a 22-member board of commissioners and later expanded to 24 members with the following representation: American Hospital Association and American Medical Association, seven seats each; American College of Physicians and American College of Surgeons, three seats each; American Dental Association, one seat; and three public members. Public members are not representatives of any consumer organizations and, unlike the other representatives on the board, who are ap-

continued

pointed by their sponsoring organization, the public members are appointed by the board itself.

JCAHO's stated purpose is to improve the quality of health care to the public.

Some 5,300 hospitals and 3,600 other health care programs are JCAHO inspected and accredited. JCAHO has programs that accredit general and psychiatric hospitals, home-care organizations, nursing homes and other long-term-care facilities. The group also has programs to accredit psychiatric services such as substance abuse programs, community mental health centers, programs for the mentally retarded, and adult and adolescent psychiatric programs. It also accredits outpatient surgery centers, urgent-care clinics, dental and other group practices, preferred provider organizations and community institutions.

JCAHO funding comes from fees charged to institutions and other programs. The organization's yearly operating budget is around $50 million.

Fewer than 1 percent of hospitals inspected by JCAHO fail to meet accreditation standards.

Over the last decade, a great deal of controversy has swirled around the organization. The People's Medical Society and other consumer groups have suggested that JCAHO is a prime example of the foxes guarding the chicken coop—typical of the health care system in the United States. A 1988 exposé in the *Wall Street Journal* raised serious questions about the credibility of the organization's inspection process. In 1990, then-Medicare-director Gail Wilensky, in testimony before the House Ways and Means Committee, noted concerns with JCAHO's hospital-accreditation program, which is used as the primary basis for deciding whether a hospital will be included in the Medicare program.

Despite these varied concerns, JCAHO remains the only technically independent body reviewing all aspects of a facility's operation.

■ Investigate the center's staff and their credentials. Call your state's licensing boards and make sure all the doctors, dentists and nurses who work there are licensed. During your get-acquainted visit to the center, ask about board certification and the specialties of the dentists and physicians on staff. As we have said before, certification does not guarantee quality care, but it is an important indicator.

Dentists who care for patients in hospital-based centers must have admitting privileges—i.e., the hospital has reviewed the dentists' education, licensing and other credentials and authorized the dentists to admit and care for their patients in the hospital and its facilities. About 40,000 dentists, specialists as well as generalists, have these privileges. If your dentist doesn't, it doesn't mean that she is not qualified. Instead, she may not treat enough patients needing hospital-based care and so may not apply for privileges. In such a case, your dentist will refer you to a dentist who has privileges.

Dentists in hospital-based centers may be on the staff full-time; they may also work there part-time and maintain a private office elsewhere; some may be volunteers as part of a rotating community service. All will have undergone the process of evaluation for admitting privileges.

Privately owned centers are staffed by a mix of dentist-owner(s) and/or paid staff dentists, many of whom are newly graduated from dental school.

You will also find dental assistants and hygienists employed in all types of dental centers.

Nurses provide a significant portion of the care in ambulatory settings, especially in surgery centers. Before any scheduled surgery, a nurse should call you to answer questions and give you final instructions to prepare for your visit. A nurse will closely monitor you in the recovery room and, using preestablished criteria, may advise your dentist on your readiness for discharge. Furthermore, a nurse should answer your questions and give you information on postoperative care, and certainly should call you the day after the surgery to check on your status.

The nursing staff should be comprised of registered nurses or nurse practitioners, permanently assigned to the outpatient center. Look for a low nurse-to-patient ratio—perhaps one nurse to every three or four surgical patients.

In an outpatient clinic at a teaching hospital, resident physicians and dentists—essentially, students-in-training—rotate through the clinic, changing every few months. Continuity of care is often assured by the nursing staff. Ask about the nursing turnover rate. A low rate is one indicator of a satisfied staff committed to outpatient care.

For successful same-day surgery without complications or the need for a hospital stay, anesthesia must be carefully and expertly given. Make sure that a board-certified anesthesiologist will administer the anesthesia and be present during the surgery. Ask to meet him before your surgery. (See chapter 3 for more on anesthesia risks.)

■ Take a look around at the equipment and atmosphere. Here you must look beyond the decorating touches to the overall cleanliness of the waiting area, examining rooms and recovery area. Are equipment, files, medications and other visible items maintained in an orderly fashion? Is the recovery room adequately equipped for the number of patients being served, and is privacy maintained? Overall, is the atmosphere professional, yet friendly? If it is a hospital-based surgery center, are the ambulatory patients treated in a separate area, with its own recovery room, staff and reception area? If not, you may be left to recover with other, more seriously ill patients and may not receive the attention you deserve.

■ Evaluate the facility's emergency preparedness. If the center is not hospital-based, ask about procedures for emergency transfer to a hospital if you should become seriously ill during or immediately after surgery. Ask how the center works with local hospitals and ambulance services. Should the need arise, can the center arrange rapid transportation to a hospital? Which hospital is used? Does the center's staff call an ambulance, and if so, which one? Do they have an emergency communication system with the hospital?

■ Find out the center's fees and billing policies. Do not assume that the fees for all services at one ambulatory center are the same as fees at others or that this is the lowest-priced alternative. Ask. Find out how payment is to be made and whether a sliding fee scale is available, if you are on a limited income. Must you pay at the time of treatment? Credit card or cash only, or can a payment schedule be arranged? What health coverage does the center accept? If you are covered by an HMO or other managed care plan, is the center part of the plan's provider network? (If not, you may have to pay most or all of the fees. Check your member's handbook or ask the plan administrator for details.)

- Find out the number of surgeries the center performs a year. More and more studies are corroborating what many people have long suspected regarding quality of surgical care: Practice makes perfect. Also ask the dentist how many times a year she performs the procedure you are about to undergo.

Ambulatory care can be convenient, safe and cost-effective, but, as with other fast-growing fields, inconsistencies in quality and service do exist. Take the time before you use the facility's services to evaluate the care you can expect.

WHEN HOSPITAL CARE IS CALLED FOR

These days, in just about every community, competition among hospitals is intense. Hospital-sponsored newsletters and advertisements tout each facility as providing comprehensive care in a high-quality, high-tech setting. But can they all be the best? How can you sift through the competing claims? What really matters when it comes to hospital care? While, admittedly, the vast majority of dental procedures and dental consumers do not require hospital-based care, nevertheless it is important to be prepared. Let's consider some of the factors.

Your Choice of Hospital

There are about 5,300 hospitals in the United States, according to the American Hospital Association. At first glance, it may seem that "a hospital is a hospital is a hospital," but the differences among the various types—community, medical center, teaching and specialty hospitals—can affect your care. Let's first look briefly at each type, then consider how to go about evaluating the care you will receive—before you need it.

COMMUNITY HOSPITALS VERSUS MEDICAL CENTERS. Community hospitals, as the name implies, dot the landscape of residential communities. They market themselves as one of your neighbors. The distinction between a community hospital and medical center is not clearly defined, however. For marketing purposes, a hospital may choose one or the other designation, so don't be fooled by the name. Both facilities may offer many of the same services, especially those related to dental surgery.

A community hospital may range from as few as 50 to as many as several hundred beds. A good-size community hospital has around 250 beds, and it offers general surgical, diagnostic, medical and often obstetrical services. It usually has every kind of high-tech medical gizmo needed to provide basic and competent care. Its operating room has the equipment necessary to perform dental surgery, although the room may be used for other surgical procedures as well. Larger community hospitals are likely to have CAT scanning, x-ray, and other diagnostic and therapeutic equipment for modern care.

If you are admitted to a small community hospital for a nondental reason and need dental care during your stay, dental services are likely to be provided on a consulting basis—that is, your physician calls in a dentist from the community who has privileges at the hospital. In larger community hospitals, one or more dentists may be employed full-time as members of the department of surgery or emergency medicine or, less commonly, of a separate department of dental medicine. Most specialists are available as consultants. If you are being admitted by your own dentist for a dental procedure, then she will provide your care whether it is a small or large community hospital.

A medical center is often (but not always) large, is affiliated with a university and offers the highest level of care, known as tertiary care. (Tertiary care frequently requires highly sophisticated technology and highly specialized practitioners in the performance of such diagnostic and therapeutic services as high-tech scanning, organ transplants, burn care, multiple-trauma care and open-heart surgery.) Its facilities may include specialized intensive-care units, a range of surgical services and an emergency department equipped to handle serious trauma victims. Medical centers argue that because of the sheer number of patients they treat, they are experienced in the care of many rare or complicated disorders. They attract well-trained specialists to their staffs and offer the latest in medical technology.

This is often true of their dental service as well. A full range of specialists are on staff full- or part-time, either in a separate department of dental medicine or as part of the department of surgery or emergency medicine. One or more operating suites are set up for dental procedures with a dental chair designed to enable the patient to be moved under sedation from a gurney to the chair. If the medical center is affiliated with a university dental teaching program, patients have 24-hour emergency access to resident dentists.

However, the characteristics of large medical centers are not always beneficial. Unless the need for such a facility is completely demonstrable, many of the attractions of such a facility may be the equivalent of a medical backfire. For example, the large size may contribute to your stress and may put policy roadblocks in the way of your active concern for your care. The greater numbers of staff, patients and visitors expose you to a greater risk of hospital-acquired infections. The presence of costly pieces of equipment makes it more likely you will undergo tests and procedures to put these devices and their technicians to work.

In the final analysis, keep in mind that a hospital's size is not always a reliable clue to the kind of treatment you can expect there. You might have a warm and caring experience at a 700-bed behemoth of a medical center, and you might be treated like yesterday's laundry at a 100-bed community hospital.

TEACHING VERSUS NONTEACHING HOSPITALS. The arguments for going to a teaching hospital are just about the same as ones for going to a medical center: expertise, the newest technology, the latest knowledge. In fact, many of the best and best-known teaching hospitals are university medical centers. About 125 of the approximately 1,500 teaching hospitals are academic medical centers, according to a report in the *American Medical News*.

There is no shortage of doctors in a teaching hospital. During a stay of even a few days, you may be seen by any or all of the following:

▪ One or more staff doctors and dentists, who are full-time employees of the hospital. They administer the hospital's teaching program, teach medical and dental students and help care for patients. Some world-renowned staff specialists may have little actual contact with most patients, except perhaps those with rare disorders. These doctors lend their prestige to the hospital and add to the overall cost of care.

- Your own community-based dentist/oral surgeon
- Your own physician, especially if you have a medical condition such as heart disease that could affect your dental health. The Joint Commission on Accreditation of Healthcare Organizations (JCAHO) requires medical supervision of dental patients in such cases.
- A resident or many residents who have their M.D., D.D.S. or D.M.D. degrees (they may or may not be licensed) and have completed an internship and are continuing postgraduate training in a specialty
- A medical or dental student or, more likely, many medical and dental students, who aren't really doctors/dentists at all but instead are in their third or fourth year of medical/dental school

Medical and dental schools place their students in university hospitals and medical centers and in affiliated community hospitals. (In fact, these hospitals exist as much for the education of medical and dental students as they do for the care of patients.) A teaching hospital has 24-hour physician coverage provided by these residents and interns, including emergency dental care. The hospital must be accredited by the Joint Commission on Accreditation of Healthcare Organizations and by the appropriate medical and dental specialty boards.

Cost may be another factor in deciding between a teaching and a nonteaching hospital. Teaching hospitals have greater expenses than nonteaching hospitals—the salaries paid to postgraduates-in-training, the money it takes to attract top-flight experts, the enormous sums paid for new technological marvels—and fewer patients at teaching hospitals pay their bills. So it's no wonder the average cost of care in a teaching hospital can be as much as twice that of a nonteaching hospital.

Evaluating a Hospital

Evaluating a hospital, like finding a qualified dentist, takes some time and research, but your efforts can pay off in better care and less anxiety and worry for you.

ACCREDITATION. At the very least, the hospital should be accredited by JCAHO. About 75 percent of hospitals have undergone these voluntary inspections, which have traditionally concerned themselves largely with procedural rather than quality issues.

What the wary consumer must keep in mind is that to seek accreditation is a voluntary act for a hospital. As with ambulatory care centers, hospitals pay for a survey, and this on-site visit is scheduled in advance, so the hospital has time to prepare and, if necessary, clean up its act. In the accrediting process, teams of investigators arrive at a hospital that has either applied for the first time or is up for renewal, which is every three years. An extensive list of items—from nursing care to hospital administration, food service to medical records—is studied and inspected to see if the standards are sufficiently high. The hospital's section or department of dental medicine must comply with the same set of standards as other departments.

The stated aim of accreditation is to set and promote high standards of quality and to reward those institutions that achieve those standards. In some cases, it may take several inspections before a hospital satisfactorily meets them. Hospitals that fail to meet standards are given an opportunity to correct the problems before another inspection.

But the seal of approval doesn't tell the whole story—accreditation procedures might uncover minor glitches in the dental operating room, but they don't always pick up major deficiencies in the humaneness of the staff or in the facility. These things you have to monitor and question for yourself.

A telephone call to the hospital's chief administrator can usually get you its accreditation status. Most hospitals post their current accreditation certificate in their lobby. Or you can contact JCAHO directly (see page 70).

One thing to keep in mind about accreditation: JCAHO approves nearly all hospitals inspected, so once again the burden remains largely on you to perform your own inspection, get your own facts and make your own assessment of the hospitals in your community.

NURSING STAFF. Nurses are the most important staff members in a hospital and certainly the professionals you face most often during a hospital stay.

People hospitalized for dental therapy are cared for along with other medical and surgical inpatients. The nurses who care for them are, in general, responsible for preventing infection, teaching the patient post-

The Nurses Who Care for You

Depending on a hospital's size and availability of nurses, you may be cared for by several levels of nursing staff.

At the top of the hierarchy are registered nurses (R.N.'s), individuals who have completed three or more years of training at a nursing school, a baccalaureate-degree program or even a master's degree course. Their training combines classroom and clinical work. On graduation, they take a national examination.

R.N.'s perform a wide range of duties under the direction of physicians and dentists, from giving injections to working with you and your dentist to prepare a plan of care for you. They may prepare and give medications, watch for signs of infection and teach you about the care you'll need after you leave the hospital. They are at or near the bedside throughout your stay, so they are more accessible to answer your questions than the dentists are likely to be.

Licensed practical nurses (L.P.N.'s) have undergone training in a state-approved program, usually lasting one year, comprising both classroom and clinical work. On completion, they must pass a national written examination. Working under the direction of R.N.'s and doctors, L.P.N.'s provide basic bedside care, including taking your temperature and other vital signs, giving injections and bathing you. In some states, they are also allowed to give medications and set up intravenous tubes, which allow you to be fed or receive drugs through your veins.

Nurses' aides (or nursing assistants) have the least training, skills and autonomy. They may complete a vocational school program or even be trained by their hospital employers. Their duties are supervised by doctors, R.N.'s and L.P.N.'s, and can range from delivering messages to bathing newborns. They may escort you to the x-ray department and take and record your vital signs.

operative care, assuring postoperative nutrition and helping the patient manage pain.

SUPPORT STAFF. In a 1990 survey by researchers from the Northwestern University Dental School of 1,755 U.S. hospitals, about one-third indicated that they had one or more dental hygienists on staff. Hospitals with 300 or more beds and those with separate departments of dental medicine were most likely to employ hygienists.

These professionals carry out many of the same tasks in hospitals that they provide in dental offices—educating patients about oral health and providing cleaning and other preventive care to medically compromised patients. For patients admitted with medical problems who develop dental problems during their hospital stay, hygienists may conduct a preliminary examination to identify the need for a dentist.

As in dental offices, dental assistants may be hired by hospitals to assist dentists—assuring that all necessary instruments and supplies are available, that the patient's dental records are on hand and that infection control procedures are carried out; and assisting during actual procedures in the operating room. Their education involves a combination of course work (see chapter 1) and on-the-job training.

HOSPITAL HAZARDS. A hospital is no place for a sick person. This is the conclusion of many experts in the medical field, but what do you do when a hospital stay is absolutely necessary? It is impossible, of course, to surround yourself with an impervious safety shield, but smart consumers arm themselves with information about where these hazards lurk and try to gain admission to hospitals where hazards are kept to a minimum.

High on the list of hazards—if not at the top—is the potential for acquiring an infection. The risk of such infections is even greater in the hospital than in your dentist's office. Nosocomial is the name given to infections acquired during hospitalization; they are produced by microorganisms that dwell with relative impunity in hospitals or arrive on the coattails of new patients. Not present in patients on admission, nosocomial infections are costly and potentially dangerous "souvenirs" of a hospital stay.

Five to 10 percent of hospitalized patients acquire hospital infections annually. So what's a concerned patient to do about these invisible invaders given that they are throughout the hospital—on the walls and floors, in the food and water, in transfused blood and intravenous fluids, perhaps even on the other bed in the room? The first line of defense comes when you're hospital-shopping. Find a hospital that has a good nosocomial record. Ask if the following elements are in place:

- At least one infection control nurse for every 250 beds
- A trained infection control physician on staff
- An active infection control committee meeting regularly
- One or more staff members who belong to the Association for Practitioners in Infection Control

Hospitals that institute an infection control program can lower their infection rate by one-third, says a Centers for Disease Control and Prevention study.

A hospital knows its infection rate, although it may be unwilling to divulge it to you. Call the local department of health or ask your doctor/dentist for the rate in the postsurgical unit. If the hospital has an active infection-control program, it keeps its physicians informed about the current rate anyway. And if you must, don't hesitate to call the hospital administrator.

YOUR EVALUATION VISIT. There are a great many factors to take into account when you are evaluating a hospital to care for you during dental surgery or other medical needs. Just remember—there is no way to know what a hospital is really like except by giving it a good once-over in person—before you become a patient.

To get the most from an on-site visit, don't just barge in, clipboard in hand and a scowl on your face. Call and ask to speak with the hospital's administrator or someone in the community relations department. Explain that you are new in town and want to see the facility because you have heard so many wonderful things about it. Tell them you may have to have some dental surgery done soon, perhaps there, and you would like to get a feel for the place. Tell them anything you think will get you in.

You will probably get a quick walk-through (if that) with some minor-level administrative employee or a hospital volunteer by your side. He will point you in all the right directions, telling you very little. Another way to get information and more than a passing glance at the place is to visit a patient and ask about the food, nursing care and other features of the hospital experience that only a patient knows firsthand. Wander around a bit, as though you belong wherever you happen to be in the building at the moment. No matter how you tour, make sure to include the postsurgical unit and emergency room.

WHERE TO GO FOR EMERGENCY CARE

If you have ever awakened in the middle of the night with a throbbing toothache, you no doubt can sympathize with the millions of Americans who seek emergency care from their dentists, clinics and hospital emergency rooms each year. While few dental conditions are life-threatening, they are nevertheless often painful, interfere with eating and generally make the sufferer miserable.

True dental emergencies, according to the American Dental Association, include a broken jaw, broken teeth with the nerve exposed, a tooth that has been knocked out, gum abscess, cuts to the cheek, severe dental pain and infection, upper airway obstruction and uncontrolled bleeding. These conditions call for care as soon as possible. By evaluating your emergency options before you need them, you help ensure fast, competent, appropriate care.

Start with your dentist. During your get-acquainted visit, ask about her emergency services:

1. **Do you have a 24-hour answering service? How are nighttime/weekend calls handled?**

2. **Typically, how quickly do you see patients with emergency needs?**

3. **Do you have times set aside each day for emergency visits?**
   A 1991 study found that dentists had an average of 14.5 emergency visits per month. To accommodate these unscheduled visits, dentists use one of two systems. The block system involves setting aside an hour

The ER as Dentist's Office

Hospital ERs are often used as outpatient clinics by families without access to private doctors or dentists. In one Seattle children's hospital, for example, the number of dental emergency visits was more than twice as large in 1991 as in 1982, according to a study published in *Pediatric Dentistry.* Yet nearly 20 percent of the children who visited as the result of dental injuries required no treatment; during the 10-year period, only four injuries were serious enough to warrant hospitalization.

Such demands seriously affect a facility's ability to provide true emergency care, can create long waits for everyone and can affect the quality of care for every patient—young and old—in the emergency-care system.

Don't be caught so unprepared that you are forced to use a crowded hospital ER when another resource would do. Instead, talk with your dentist about where to go and when to call her in an emergency. Look at alternatives to the ER in your community, such as walk-in dental centers.

in the morning and one in the afternoon during which emergency visits are scheduled. This system, often used in new practices with fewer regular patients, provides some reassurance that you will be seen promptly and with minimal waiting. Busier practices often prefer to "fit you in," using cancellations or time when the dentist is waiting for anesthesia to take effect or the hygienist is with another patient. Such a system is a balancing act, calling for a skilled scheduling assistant/receptionist to prevent long waits or rushed care.

4. Do you ever refer patients to the hospital for emergency care? Which one(s)? Why?

The authors of a Baltimore study published in the *Journal of the American Dental Association* in 1996 concluded that "hospital emergency departments are not the most appropriate setting for treatment when dental emergencies occur." They point out that the care is costly and less likely to be definitive than that provided in dental offices. In fact, many community hospitals are not staffed or equipped to handle dental emergencies. Hospitals affiliated with dental schools and major medical centers are most likely to have dentists and dental residents on call at all times. However, even this doesn't guarantee you'll be seen by a dentist. The authors of the Baltimore study found that while the teaching hospital they examined had a fully staffed dentistry department, dental emergencies were rarely referred to it. Care, which primarily consisted of prescriptions for pain medication or antibiotics, was provided by the doctors in the emergency room.

There may be some occasions when you'll have few options other than the emergency room—it's midnight and the bleeding from an earlier extraction won't stop; your daughter has just lost a tooth in a Sunday afternoon soccer game; you've developed a fever and swelling in your lower jaw while your dentist is out of town. So just in case, ask your dentist about hospital emergency care in your community. Then do some checking on your own.

A 1992 report on emergency care published in *U.S. News & World Report* suggests that you write to prospective hospitals' quality-assurance representatives or emergency department chiefs and ask the following questions:

1. **What is the proportion of part-time (or moonlighting) doctors to full-time emergency physicians?**

2. **What proportion of patients make an unplanned return visit for the same problem within 72 hours?**

3. **How many times during the past three months has a discrepancy between an emergency room doctor's reading of x-ray reports and a radiologist's interpretations required a patient to return to see a specialist?**

The written response should come back with low numbers in each case for the best overall emergency rooms.

In addition, when you tour and evaluate local hospitals, make sure you visit the emergency facilities and ask to talk with the department administrator or head nurse. Among the questions to ask are the following:

1. Does the department's staff include any or all of the following practitioners: emergency physician, oral and maxillofacial surgeon, periodontist, pediatric dentist, general dentist? Is there 24-hour coverage?

2. Does the department have one or more trauma rooms, and is at least one equipped for dental care?

3. How many dental emergencies are treated in the department each year?

4. What is the nurse turnover rate (a clue to staff burnout and dissatisfaction)?

5. Is a quality-assurance program in place to monitor how well the department cares for its patients?

6. Are one or more social workers assigned to the department?

7. Is two-way communication available with local ambulances?

Let's return to the setting where most people receive their dental care—the dental office.

3

When You Visit

 ou've interviewed several dentists and visited their offices. Based on your survey, you've selected a dentist. Now, it's time to put your selection to the test. Ideally, your first visit as a new patient will be for preventive care, rather than for an emergency. So let's look at what you can expect during your *first* preventive visit. Recall visits, also called maintenance visits, and emergencies are covered later in this chapter.

AN OUNCE OF PREVENTION

When you visit a general dentist for the first time, you should expect to have three things happen. First, you will be asked to complete a thorough patient history. Second, the dentist will carry out a complete examination. Finally, your teeth will be cleaned. (Sometimes the second and third steps are reversed, depending upon the individual dentist's practice.) Dental hygienists are trained to perform each of these tasks, and may do so, depending on your state's dental practice laws, but commonly a dentist will do at least some of them. If your dentist is among the 30 to 40 percent of general dentists who don't have a dental hygienist on staff, then the dentist will perform all parts. Let's look at each one in detail.

Patient History

As we mentioned in the previous chapter, a complete medical and dental history can be a valuable tool to protect you from infection and dental complications. It also serves several other purposes as well, including:

- Identifying potential dental conditions such as old fillings that must be evaluated during your current examination
- Identifying possible medical conditions such as diabetes that have been previously unrecognized and may need referral to a physician
- Documenting past and present dental care as a baseline for planning and carrying out future care
- Assessing your general health and nutritional status because physical and mental disabilities may affect your ability to carry out dental care at home; poor eating habits may contribute to decay and other oral diseases

The patient history may include both a written questionnaire and an oral interview. When you call for your first appointment, the receptionist may ask several preliminary questions beyond your name and that of your insurance company.

1. **Are you currently taking any prescription or over-the-counter medications?**

   If you are taking anticoagulants ("blood thinners"), for example, your dentist may want to call your physician before your appointment to discuss any potential bleeding problems.

2. **Have you had rheumatic fever, heart valve replacement or hip replacement surgery?**

   Whenever procedures that cause bleeding are performed, people with these conditions are at risk for bacteremia (bacteria in the blood) and subsequent infections. Root planing is such a procedure and is part of the basic cleaning that is done. To lessen the risk, your dentist may prescribe an antibiotic to be taken before your visit.

   Your dentist may mail the patient history form to you before your visit so you can complete it in private and with access to any personal records you might keep about your medical and dental health. The more accurate it is, the less the likelihood that you or the dentist will face unpleasant surprises from complications or allergic reactions.

More typically, you will be asked to complete the questionnaire in the dentist's reception area once you've arrived for your visit. In such cases, you'll want to have available information on the following:

- Your history of major illnesses and surgeries. Chronic illnesses such as leukemia and lupus can make a patient more susceptible to infection. A history of problems with postsurgical healing could influence any recommendations for oral surgery.

- Current prescription and over-the-counter medications. These can be important for two reasons. First, some drugs cause problems with teeth and gums that may need dental care. For example, phenytoin (Dilantin), which is prescribed for epileptic seizures, headaches, heart conditions and some other conditions, causes enlargement of the gums. If the swelling is left untreated, bacteria collect under the gums and cause severe infections. The inflammation can even force teeth to move out of position. The second reason dentists need to know about the drugs you are taking is to avoid drug interactions and overdoses with those they might prescribe or use during procedures.

- Allergies to any medications, not just those used previously in dental procedures, and to foods, which could affect dietary recommendations the dentist might make

- The names of your physician(s) and other health care providers, in case your dentist needs to consult prior to performing a procedure

- Your history of recent dental care, including the most recent x-rays taken, anesthesia used and procedures carried out. The dentist can request a copy of your records from your previous dentist, but your recollection is useful also.

- The name(s) of dental specialists you are consulting

- The history of injuries to your mouth, jaw or teeth. Scars and decreased function could complicate procedures or inhibit your ability to carry out home dental care effectively.

- The current problem, if any, that prompted the dental appointment
- Your use of alcohol and tobacco

- Your home dental care activities, including the frequency of flossing, brushing and using mouth rinses

Once you've completed the questionnaire, you will be escorted into either the dentist's office/consultation room or the operatory. Before carrying out any procedure, even an examination, the dentist needs to review your history and clarify items you were unsure of or get more information than the form allowed. You may also have questions or concerns that you've thought of since your get-acquainted visit. This is a good opportunity to ask them before the dentist starts picking and probing.

This is also an ideal time to bring up your fears or previous bad experiences with dentistry. While an examination is unlikely to be painful, it is nevertheless a good idea to put your fears on the table from the beginning. If you haven't visited a dentist for some time, you may not be aware of the range of techniques now available to make dentistry practically painless and to calm patients' anxiety, as we describe later in this chapter. Only when you make the dentist aware of your fears can he suggest ways to calm them.

If the conversation to this point hasn't touched on any specific oral health concerns you have, mention them now before you get distracted by the bright light in your face and probes against your gums.

Physical Examination

You will be seated in the dental chair for this second stage, the full dental examination. The dentist wears latex gloves, a surgical mask and protective glasses. The assistant puts a disposable bib around your neck, reclines the chair and directs the overhead light onto your face.

During your first visit to a new dentist, the comprehensive examination proceeds in phases, working from the outside to the inside. The dentist looks closely at the skin on your face and neck, then uses his fingertips to feel your lymph nodes under your chin and along your neck. Standing behind you, he lays two fingers on each side of your face at the joint of your upper and lower jaw. When you open and close your mouth, he can assess your jaw function. Abnormalities may affect your ability to eat, carry out home dental care and undergo dental procedures comfortably. Problems with this joint can also cause headaches and/or facial pain associated with temporomandibular disorder, or TMD (also

Taking Control of Your Fears

According to the American Dental Association (ADA), about 12 million Americans are so dental phobic that they avoid going to dentists except when severe pain or another dental emergency forces them into the dental chair. Many others experience varying degrees of dental anxiety. If you are among them, discussing your fears with your dentist can open the way to a range of available techniques. Some common methods:

■ Distraction techniques using video games, films, headphones with music or aquariums. The goal is to focus your attention on something other than the dental procedure.

■ Relaxation techniques such as hypnosis or audiotapes that take you through a series of total body relaxation exercises. The ADA estimates that about 20 percent of dentists are trained to apply hypnosis for deep relaxation.

■ Aromatherapy. Researchers at Case Western Reserve University found that 82 percent of dental patients experienced less anxiety when a floral fragrance was used in the office during their procedures.

■ Paced therapy, in which the dentist carries out only one phase of therapy at each visit, starting with the least likely to cause pain or anxiety and slowly building to the stages requiring anesthesia. Throughout the visits, the dentist explains before proceeding what will take place, if any discomfort is to be expected and how long the procedure should take.

■ Prearranged signals. Having discussed your fear with the dentist, you can agree that when you need a break or if you feel pain, you will signal and the dentist will immediately stop. This technique is particularly effective for those patients who fear loss of control more than they fear pain.

■ Demonstrations and simulations, in which the dentist uses a model to show you the current ways in which a procedure is carried out. Many adults' fears developed years ago when drills were slower and anesthetics were less effective.

called temporomandibular joint disorder, or TMJ), which we discuss in chapter 7.

The assessment now concentrates on your mouth. The dentist examines your tongue, top and bottom; the inner lining of your cheeks; your lips, inside and outside; and your palate. This examination may include not only looking at each structure closely, but also feeling it and taking measurements of any sores, lumps or irregularities.

Tools of the Trade

Nearly all the tools used by a general dentist fit onto a tray about 12 inches long and 8 inches wide. This tray commonly sits alongside you and the dentist while he works. If you look closely during an examination, you are likely to find the following:

- A small, round, long-handled mirror for viewing the inside of your mouth
- One or more pointed probes, called explorers, for examining tooth crevices, between teeth and so on
- A periodontal probe with calibrated markings along the working end to measure the depth of the space between the tooth and gum (called pockets)
- A scaler (looking rather like a tiny garden hoe) and other handheld instruments used to scrape plaque from teeth and their roots
- Tweezers
- A handpiece with its various heads (removable heads for cleaning, drilling and other procedures that are fastened to the handpiece—popularly called a drill—which is attached by tubes or cords to a power source)
- Cotton rolls
- A disposable tray mat on which all items lie

Other items, such as heads for removing decay prior to filling teeth, tiny round files for carrying out root canal therapy or a syringe for administering anesthetic, may be added if needed.

As he proceeds, the dentist either logs his findings directly in your medical record or dictates them for his assistant to transcribe. The charts he uses to record his findings have illustrations of the parts of the mouth, which make it simple for the dentist to note the location of scars, lumps or other findings.

Your gums are next. The dentist gently pulls your cheeks and lips outward to see the full gum. In particular, he's looking for a good, even pink color; a snug fit around your teeth; a firm consistency with a smooth surface below the tooth line and a slightly rough surface near the tooth; and an absence of swelling, pus or bleeding. Using a periodontal probe, he will slide the tip of the probe into the small space between a tooth and the surrounding gum. The probe's calibrated tip allows for easy depth measurement (the deeper the gap, the greater the likelihood of periodontal disease).

Finally, he examines your teeth, using various explorers to pick at the edges of fillings, crevices of molars and spots on teeth that may indicate cavities or worn enamel. He also scrapes the teeth, especially along the gum line and on the vertical surfaces, to evaluate how much plaque and calculus (hardened plaque) are present. He records any potential problems in your record using a standardized numbered tooth system.

Throughout this process, the dentist may chatter about the weather, work in silence or explain what's happening at each step. It's largely up to you. Not every patient wants to hear the details, so the dentist will probably wait for your cue. As an alert medical consumer, however, you know the value of keeping informed. Ask him to describe what he is doing and why. Don't hesitate to interrupt the examination if you have questions.

Aids in Your Examination

X-RAYS. Unless you have had a full set of bitewing x-rays done within the past five to eight years, the dentist will want to take them at some point during your examination. You can avoid unnecessary exposure by having the dentist request a set of these recent x-rays from your previous dentist. You will have to wait until they are received before getting your treatment plan, but the fewer x-rays, the better.

During your earlier get-acquainted visit, as we described in chapter 2, you examined the office procedures for taking x-rays. If you now find differences in how your x-rays are actually taken, stop the process and ask why. Remember, for example, that you should be covered by a lead apron and collar.

X-rays provide a baseline for comparison to detect future changes in your teeth and bone and reveal conditions within these structures that can be detected no other way. The Food and Drug Administration guidelines recommend that dentists take a series of bitewing x-rays. These x-ray films show the crown and part of the root for two or three pairs (upper and lower) of teeth. Bitewing x-rays are especially valuable in detecting decay between teeth. For the initial examination, four to five bitewings give a full view.

The dentist (or hygienist) inserts a small rectangle of x-ray film into a T-shaped plastic or Styrofoam holder. She asks you to rinse with a bacteria-killing mouth rinse. With you sitting in an upright position, she inserts the film and holder into your mouth, pressing the film against your palate and inner gum line without bending it. She asks you to bite together, with one "leg" of the holder between your teeth. Positioning the x-ray tube next to your cheek, she steps behind a protective screen and takes the x-ray. This process is repeated to give full views of your side and back teeth, then the arm of the x-ray machine is moved out of the way once again and the film is developed in the office's darkroom, usually by the dental assistant or hygienist.

If during the examination the dentist finds suspicious features such as tooth discoloration or signs of gum disease, then periapical films should also be taken of the involved teeth. In a process similar to that for bitewings, periapical x-ray films show side views of up to four teeth per film from root tip to crown top and provide information on how well the teeth are sitting in the sockets. These x-rays also show any bone damage or loss.

CASTS. The dentist may also suggest that he make study casts of your teeth, especially if your teeth are poorly aligned or appear to need extensive dental work. Casts are life-size plaster or stone reproductions of your upper and lower teeth and gums. The casts show the present condition of your mouth and, as such, are especially valuable for patients about to undergo orthodontic, cosmetic or extensive restoration work. Casts show wear patterns, the effects of missing or misaligned teeth, the position and size of your gums and, of course, tooth positions. Casts also can be an effective communication tool for the dentist to explain proposed treatments or for you to describe problem areas.

To prepare for cast-making, the dentist asks you to rinse vigorously, use dental floss to remove food or other debris, then rinse with a mouth rinse. Using a cotton roll or compressed air, he dries your teeth and gums. The plastic impression trays come in several sizes, so he inserts empty ones until he has the right fit. He fills a tray with the special paste, inserts it quickly over your lower teeth under your tongue and presses firmly for three minutes until the paste sets. After rinsing again, you have the same procedure done for your upper teeth.

From these impressions, a laboratory technician, hygienist or assistant makes the cast using plaster of Paris or dental stone. The casts become part of your dental record.

LABORATORY TESTS. The chances are good that you will complete your examination without any tests beyond x-rays—not something that can be said for many medical examinations. Laboratory tests are the exception rather than the rule in dental care. Nevertheless, you don't want to undergo them unquestioningly.

The most common tests are the cytologic smear and the biopsy. The cytologic smear technique removes surface cells for examination. A suspicious area is scraped with a small, flexible metal spatula, and the sample is smeared onto a glass slide, which is sent to a laboratory for analysis. Smears are used to identify herpesviruses or *Candida albicans* fungus or to establish if radiation therapy has been successful in treating oral cancer.

Cytologic smears have limited value for several reasons. The procedure can be used to test only surface conditions, not deep growths. In addition, the results are not sufficiently reliable to base treatment on in many cases. False-negative results—indicating that no disease is present when in fact it is—are common enough that a biopsy may still need to be performed. Even positive smears do not provide enough specific information to implement treatment, except in the case of *Candida* infections. Thus, a biopsy may also be necessary to rule out a false-positive finding (indicating disease is present when it isn't) or, in the case of a true positive, to provide details about the kind of cells present and how much tissue is involved.

Biopsies are performed when growths, white patches or dark pigmented areas inside the cheek or on other normally pink oral areas are detected. Only about 7 percent of all cancers occur in or around the mouth, but when detected early and treated, oral cancer is usually curable. However, its signs are very similar to those of other less serious conditions, and only a biopsy can effectively differentiate.

Your dentist may perform the biopsy or refer you to a specialist. For small growths, the entire area may be cut out under local anesthesia; only a portion of a larger tumor is removed for testing. Samples of the tissue are examined under a microscope to detect cancer cells.

Another set of circumstances may lead your dentist to order various basic laboratory tests such as urinalysis and a white blood cell count. Some diseases—AIDS, leukemia, diabetes and sickle-cell anemia, among them—affect the gums, lymph nodes, tongue and other areas of the mouth and jaw. An alert dentist may be the first to spot these symptoms. It is then appropriate to suggest laboratory tests to diagnose the suspected illness and to refer you to a physician.

While none of the tests used in dentistry carries significant risk, you should nevertheless ask questions before agreeing to any test. In particular, you want to know:

1. **What is the test called? How exactly is it performed?**

2. **What do you expect the test to show?**

3. **Why is the test necessary?**

4. **Will it hurt? Are there any risks?**

5. **Will you perform it? Who analyzes the results?**

6. **Can I get a copy of the test results?**

7. **How long will the test take? How long before the results are known?**

8. How much does it cost? Do I have to get preapproval from my HMO or insurance company to ensure coverage?

9. What happens if I do not undergo the test? Are there any alternatives?

10. Do the potential benefits outweigh the risks?

Treatment Plan

The ultimate goals of the history, examination, x-rays, laboratory tests and casts are to establish your current oral health, highlight potential medical and dental problems and suggest one or more resolutions. Once all the stages of this first preventive examination are complete, your new dentist should discuss the findings and present your treatment plan. This can usually be done during your initial visit, but may be delayed to a second visit if extensive work is anticipated that would need time and cost estimates to be developed; if x-rays are coming from your previous dentist; if test results are awaited from an outside laboratory; or if the dentist wants to consult your physician or dental specialists. (Of course, if you have no dental problems, you won't need a treatment plan beyond the recommendation for a cleaning and regular maintenance visits.)

As we said in chapter 1, a treatment plan should answer the following questions:

1. What problems have been identified?

2. What treatment alternatives are available?

3. What are the advantages and disadvantages of each?

4. What are the risks attached to each alternative?

5. What is the probable outcome of treatment?

6. What is the cost of each alternative?

7. How much time is needed?

8. What are the consequences of doing nothing at this time?

About 40 percent of adults need dental treatment beyond routine maintenance at any given time. If your oral health is good and only a filling or two is needed, the dentist may simply tell you the treatment plan. If you want it in writing, ask for it. For more extensive work, especially if it involves several appointments for a series of procedures, the dentist will probably write up a plan. Insist on one if he doesn't and make sure it answers the questions listed above. Since there may be a lot of information to consider, perhaps even options, you do not have to decide during this visit. A written plan allows you to consider all the alternatives, discuss them with family or health care providers and, if necessary, begin investigating financial arrangements. (For information on some of the procedures commonly included in treatment plans, see chapter 4.)

Cleaning

Whatever lies ahead of you in the way of treatment, one thing is certain: Your first preventive visit to a new dentist ends with a professional cleaning. (If your history and examination have taken most of your appointment time, you may need to schedule a second appointment for a thorough cleaning.)

A comprehensive cleaning, known as oral prophylaxis, helps prevent gum disease by removing plaque and calculus from teeth above the gum line with a procedure known as scaling and below the gum line with root planing. Just how much scaling and root planing you undergo is determined by the degree of gum disease that is apparent. Patients with gingivitis—inflammation of the gums with some redness or swelling caused by infection—are likely to undergo scaling, perhaps with a topical anesthetic to numb the gum's surface nerve endings or a new-on-the-scene gel applied to the teeth to soften the calculus, making the scaling easier and potentially less painful. If the infection has started to spread to the underlying bone and the gums are pulling away from the teeth—which constitutes a condition known as periodontitis—root planing is added to the process. A local anesthetic, which is popularly called novocaine but which in fact is lidocaine or another similar drug, given by injection will deaden the nerves deep within the gum. Deeper root planing is applied for periodontitis that involves so much bone damage that teeth are loose in their sockets. (See chapter 6 for more on the treatment of periodontitis.)

The dentist (or hygienist) starts the cleaning process by removing debris on and around your teeth with compressed air, water, floss and bacterial mouth rinses. Then she uses the scalers and planers to manually scrape plaque and calculus from each tooth. She moves these tiny hoelike or sicklelike instruments in an upward scraping motion around the vertical surfaces of your teeth. To complete the root planing, she slides the planer gently below the gum line and again scrapes upward. By so doing, she smooths the outside wall of the root, which allows the gum to once again attach to the tooth.

She follows by polishing your teeth with a mild abrasive paste applied with a small rubber cup attachment to her handpiece. Polishing removes stains but has an important preventive function as well: Plaque doesn't stick well to a smooth tooth surface.

People with healthy gums and clean teeth may be offered topical fluoride—i.e., fluoride that is applied to the surface of the teeth—as the final step in cleaning. While the benefits of fluoride are greatest in newly erupted teeth, even adult teeth will absorb fluoride, resulting in remineralization of spots that could become cavities if left untreated. In particular, individuals who live in communities without fluoridated water

Removing Plaque With Sound Waves

Ultrasonic scaling devices use very high frequency sound waves in the form of rapid vibrations (up to 42,000 cycles per second) to remove plaque and calculus from your teeth. The dentist (or hygienist) moves the tip of the handheld device lightly several times across the surface of each tooth. You hear a shrill whine from the air turbine that operates the device, but you don't feel the heat generated because a very fine water spray helps to cool the tip and wash away debris. The dentist finishes the process by manually removing plaque in areas that could not be reached with the ultrasonic device.

continued

Ultrasonic scaling will usually be faster than manual scaling and involves less injury to gum tissues and little or no pain. The water spray lessens visibility for the dentist, however, and both you and the dentist can quickly become soaked by the mist. You need protection for your eyes and clothes; a saliva ejector (the tube that draws water and saliva from your mouth); and frequent stops to spit and dry off.

Perhaps more important, if the tip is not kept moving, the heat being generated by the waves can damage the inner structure of your tooth. Ultrasonic scaling is also not recommended for certain groups of people:

- People with increased susceptibility to infection or respiratory disease. The water spray becomes contaminated with bacteria from their mouths and can be breathed into the lungs.

- People with cardiac pacemakers. The magnetic field produced by the device can interfere with pacemaker function.

- Children. Their still-developing tissues are sensitive to the vibrations, and their new teeth are particularly vulnerable to the heat generated.

- People with areas of tooth surface worn away

- People with porcelain crowns, which can be broken by the vibrations; composite resin fillings, which can have the surface veneer removed by the procedure; and titanium implants for permanent dentures, which can be damaged

- People with very little accumulation of calculus between dental visits

Before the dentist begins the process, ask how long she has been using the device, what training she has had and why she is using ultrasonic rather than manual scaling. Remind her of any aspects of your medical history that could affect the outcome. If you have any doubts about your suitability or the dentist's expertise, ask her to carry out manual scaling.

can benefit from a regular program of topical fluoride applied by either themselves or their dentists or through toothpastes and even fluoride tablets. For more on the benefits of and concerns about fluoride and application options, see chapter 5.

You will leave this first visit to your new dentist with more than smooth, clean teeth and perhaps a new toothbrush. You will have made an initial assessment of the skill and professionalism of your new dentist and his staff. You will be armed with essential information about your future dental needs and what you can do to maintain your oral health—including regular maintenance visits. The question now is: When should you go back?

PREVENTIVE MAINTENANCE FOR YOUR TEETH

Traditionally, the American Dental Association (ADA) and most dentists have recommended visiting your dentist every six months for a maintenance, or recall, examination and cleaning. In recent years, however, dental researchers have begun advocating a more individual approach, based on your level of risk of oral disease. In a 1995 *American Journal of Dentistry* article, Judith A. Jones, D.D.S., M.P.H., asserts that it is possible to identify people who are at low, moderate and high risk of developing root cavities. Low-risk patients, those who have had no new or repeat cavities in the past three years, need only annual checkups, according to her schedule. Moderate-risk patients are those with one or two new or repeat cavities over the past three years or with significant root surface exposed. These patients should visit their dentists every six months. Finally, high-risk patients have had three or more root cavities within the past three years and need quarterly visits and treatment.

So if your dentist suggests a regular six-month recall visit, ask why he does so. If you show moderate or extensive plaque buildup, experience signs of periodontal disease such as deep pockets around the base of your teeth or have symptoms such as pain or tooth sensitivity to heat or cold, then you probably need to make maintenance visits at least every six months. If, on the other hand, you and your dentist agree that you are at low risk for cavities, periodontal disease or other dental problems, then every 12 to 18 months may be adequate unless your health changes.

These recall visits are a modified version of your first preventive visit. In particular, during recall visits, the dentist checks for tooth color changes that can mean cavities; signs of periodontal disease; and fillings that are loose, chipped or developing decay at the edges. If he identifies problems such as these, he may take one or more bitewing x-rays. If the problem is confirmed by the x-ray, he outlines the treatment plan. Before you leave, your teeth are scraped to remove the plaque and polished with mild abrasive paste.

A FEW MORE WORDS ON INFECTION CONTROL

The normal healthy human mouth can contain more than 40 different types of bacteria, viruses and fungi. Little wonder then that the 890-page textbook *Clinical Practice of the Dental Hygienist* devotes three of its first four chapters to infection and its control.

In 1993, in its recommendations for infection control practices for dentistry, the Centers for Disease Control and Prevention listed the following microorganisms as potentially found in dental offices:

- Cytomegalovirus
- Hepatitis B virus
- Hepatitis C virus
- Herpes simplex virus types 1 and 2
- Human immunodeficiency virus (HIV)
- Mycobacterium tuberculosis
- Staphylococci
- Streptococci
- Various other upper respiratory tract viruses and bacteria

As we discussed in chapter 2, among the ways disease can potentially be spread in dental offices are contaminated instruments, equipment or surfaces such as dental chair arms; airborne droplets from water spray or dental workers; and direct contact with blood, saliva or other body fluids from other patients or dental workers.

The level of risk to patients has not been definitively identified. Only when clusters of infection occur is a connection to a specific dentist usually made. When individual patients become ill several days or weeks after a dental visit, such a connection is not made. Studies have found that 34 to 68 percent of water samples from high-speed drills and air-water syringes contain various types of *Legionella* bacteria, including those that cause Legionnaires' disease and its milder form, Pontiac fever. No outbreaks of Legionnaires' disease have been traced to dental offices to date, however, and the flulike symptoms of Pontiac fever often go unreported or misdiagnosed. Thus, the potential for infection is real, but no one—from the experts at the Centers for Disease Control and Prevention to patients—can put a number on it.

Nevertheless, there are precautions that both you and your dentist *can* and *should* take. As we emphasized in chapter 2, you take control of the situation by asking about the dentist's infection control procedures during your get-acquainted visit and reinforcing your concern at each office visit. Also:

■ Insist that the dentist and anyone working with him at chairside wear fresh latex gloves (after washing their hands) and face mask.

■ Because individuals with weakened immune systems are more susceptible to infection, reschedule any dental work if you are ill.

■ Above all, be observant and ask questions if you have any doubt that proper infection control procedures are being followed.

For example, all instruments that come into contact with the inside of your mouth must be sterilized after each use or disposed of. The most effective routine is to preclean the instruments by soaking them in a mild disinfectant solution, cleaning them either manually or in an ultrasonic cleaning device, and then packaging and sterilizing them with steam heat, dry heat or chemicals. The instruments are then stored in their packaging and, just prior to use, removed and arranged on the dental tray.

Surfaces such as the handles of faucets and equipment operated during your procedure—for example, x-ray equipment or the overhead light—should be wrapped with disposable foil or plastic that is replaced between patients. Other surfaces such as countertops should be wiped with a bleach or other disinfectant solution between patients.

Repeated studies that find high levels of bacteria in water coming from high-speed drills, air-water syringes and other water-cooled devices have drawn considerable attention to finding ways to effectively eliminate this potential hazard. Using a self-contained sterile water supply has been tried by some, but researchers have found that unless scrupulous disinfecting according to the manufacturer's instructions is followed, hoses quickly become contaminated, and so does the water that passes through them. Others have suggested running handpieces two minutes at the start of the day and 20 to 30 seconds between each patient to flush the system. While this has some immediate effect, it does nothing to rid the hoses of the bacteria clinging to their walls, so the hygienic effect seems to be short-lived. Nevertheless, until more effective techniques are found, your dentist should include the flushing technique in his infection control protocols.

WHAT ABOUT PAIN?

Unlike medicine's drug cabinet, dentistry's list of appropriate and efficacious drugs is relatively small. From the patient's perspective, probably the most important medications are those to prevent or eliminate pain associated with dental procedures ranging from cleanings to oral surgery.

For thousands of years, patients had to accept pain as an inevitable part of dentistry. With the discovery of the sedative nitrous oxide in 1844 and the local anesthetic Novocain in 1904, relatively painless dentistry became a reality—for people who could afford it. Until the mid-1930s, injections of Novocain were elective, with a separate fee that left many patients to face the pain stoically—or any way they could. However, once dentists recognized the competitive advantages of being a "painless dentist" and the improved working conditions in carrying out procedures on patients who were less stressed, less anxious and not in need of restraint, Novocain became an accepted tool of practice with almost all patients.

Today, several levels of pain control and sedation are applied, depending on your tolerance of pain, your level of anxiety and the type of procedure.

■ Topical anesthetic is now available in several forms, including a patch similar to an adhesive bandage, a gel usually applied with a cotton swab, and a spray. Affecting the nerve cells immediately below the surface of your gums, it is short-acting and numbs only the immediate vicinity of application. It is commonly used to lessen discomfort during scaling and prior to injection of local anesthetic.

- Local anesthetics are the most widely used form of anesthesia in dentistry. As we mentioned earlier, today's local anesthetics, which are popularly referred to as novocaine, are more likely to be newer drugs such as lidocaine, mepivacaine or prilocaine. Injected through a thin, hollow needle into your gum, local anesthetics work on the nerves to block pain impulses to the brain. The effect, which typically comes on within three to five minutes, occurs only within the immediate vicinity of the injection.

- General anesthesia, produced by either injection or inhalation, produces unconsciousness. Its use is primarily reserved for major oral procedures such as reconstructive surgery or for patients with cerebral palsy or other conditions that prevent them from quietly sitting during extensive treatment. It may also be used for extremely anxious patients undergoing several hours of therapy. Finally, if a serious infection with swelling is present, local anesthesia may be ineffective, so general anesthesia may be necessary to carry out needed treatment.

Topical and local anesthetics carry few risks. At one time fainting was fairly common following anesthesia injection. In response to the stress of the injection and the anesthetic, the body's reflexes reduced the amount of blood flowing from the heart and, thus, to the brain, causing the patient to pass out. However, dentists found that putting the patient in a reclining position during the injection lets the blood flow more easily to the brain. Allergic reactions to topical anesthetics include a skin rash or swelling near the site of use; people may also react to an overdose with temporarily elevated blood pressure, pulse rate and breathing rate. Local anesthetic injected too close to the optic nerve can cause blurred or double vision. If the injection strikes a facial nerve, you might experience drooping of your mouth or difficulty closing your eyelid. Fortunately, all these side effects are temporary, lasting only until the anesthetic effect wears off.

As you might suspect, general anesthesia, involving loss of consciousness, carries greater risk than local. The anesthesia affects your survival reflexes, including the gag reflex, leaving you vulnerable to inadvertently swallowing dental debris or inhaling fluid into your lungs. Your breathing may have to be mechanically assisted if you are undergoing a lengthy procedure under deep general anesthesia. Should you

Pain Relief Without Drugs

If you are among the less than 1 percent of dental patients who are allergic to local anesthetics or for whom the sight of the syringe brings on panic, you may want to ask your dentist about several drug-free alternatives. Acupuncture, hypnosis and electronic dental anesthesia are effective in some patients for some types of procedures.

Acupuncture involves applying tiny, thin needles to one area of the body in order to anesthetize another part. Specifically, to achieve anesthesia in the mouth, the needle is inserted into the muscle between your thumb and forefinger. Patients feel a tingling and numbness at the site of the acupuncture needle, but no pain.

Hypnosis has been known to produce not only relaxation but also the effect of local anesthesia. Inducing a state of conscious sedation (see page 108), the dentist then uses verbal suggestion to bring about numbness in the area to be treated. Dentists at Tel Aviv University have described patients who have undergone fillings, root canal therapy and even tooth extractions while under hypnosis.

Electronic dental anesthesia devices apply a weak electrical current through patches attached with adhesive to a person's cheeks. The patient or the dentist adjusts the current level until an effective level of painlessness is achieved and continues to adjust it throughout the procedure.

None of these techniques works for all people or all procedures. The electronic device, for example, works best for procedures near the surface of teeth and gums and for the upper teeth in the front. Hypnosis requires a high level of trust between the patient and the dentist; not all people can successfully be hypnotized. While none of these techniques is painful or carries significant side effects, they are not without their

continued

problems. People afraid of needles are not likely to respond to acupuncture. Rarely, people under hypnosis experience serious psychological effects unrelated to the dental procedure. In some people, the use of the electronic device causes facial muscle twitching, and the vibrations that accompany the device's use seem to be more uncomfortable than a shot of local anesthetic.

Nevertheless, if your physician has advised you to avoid local anesthesia because of allergies, asthma or other medical problems, or if you have decided that you must have a needle-less way to achieve pain control, ask your dentist which of these options might be appropriate. Be sure that he is trained and experienced in the use of the procedure you select or has experienced practitioners on his staff.

fail to get enough oxygen for even a few minutes during the procedure, you could suffer brain damage or even death. Fortunately, not all potential complications of general anesthesia are so severe: People often complain of sore throat, headaches, nausea, dizziness and heart palpitations following procedures performed under general anesthesia. Injury to the temporomandibular joint may occur as the dentist pulls your mouth open too wide or keeps it open too long because you are unable to express any discomfort.

As we have described above, few circumstances call for general anesthesia. Most experts agree, moreover, that procedures requiring general anesthesia are best performed in a hospital, outpatient surgery center or comparably equipped specialist's office.

To protect yourself from becoming a victim of even temporary side effects, do your homework. Before you undergo any anesthesia, ask what drug is being used. If you have had previous allergic reactions to or side effects with the drug, discuss these with the dentist before anesthesia is given. Don't assume that the dentist will have checked your history.

Confirm that the person administering the anesthesia is trained and licensed to do so. Only Colorado allows a dental hygienist to administer local anesthesia without the presence in the office of a dentist. Twenty-one other states permit hygienists to give injections for local anesthesia but only with a dentist present. All states regulate anyone administering general anesthesia, requiring proof of training and application for a permit. The law may not require the dentist to display the permit, so ask to see it.

Reassure yourself that the office is equipped and the staff are trained to handle an emergency (see chapter 2), should it arise during the procedure, including at least one person present who knows cardiopulmonary resuscitation (CPR).

THE ROLE OF SEDATIVES

It isn't necessary for a drug to eliminate the sensation of pain in order to produce the effect of painless dentistry. The various sedatives used in dentistry work their magic by tricking your brain into perceiving pain as much less than it is.

People who are especially anxious about having dental work done may be given a mild sedative to take just before their dental visit. If a long procedure is planned, the dentist may inject a sedative, as well as a local anesthetic, to lessen body tension and anxiety. This form of sedation, known as conscious sedation, leaves you awake and able to speak.

Another way to achieve conscious sedation is with nitrous oxide, commonly referred to as "laughing gas," which is administered as a gas mixed with oxygen via an anesthetic mask. According to a survey by the ADA, use of nitrous oxide rose from 35 percent of dentists in 1983 to 58 percent in 1991. Among pediatric dentists, the use is even higher, with 88 percent of dentists reporting use with young patients.

Among the sedatives currently in use in dentistry are the following:

- Barbiturates such as pentobarbital (Nembutal)
- Hypnotics such as chloral hydrate
- Minor tranquilizers, including diazepam (Valium)
- Narcotics such as meperidine (Demerol)
- Antihistamines, including diphenhydramine (Benadryl)
- Ketamine, a dissociative drug that makes you feel detached from your surroundings

These medications are usually given orally, especially if only a small dose is being given before a filling or other routine dental procedure. If you are undergoing a longer procedure—for example, having several teeth extracted—the dentist may give the sedative by intravenous injection. In this, a needle connected to a tube is inserted in a vein in your hand and the sedative slowly injected.

As with dental anesthesia, sedatives carry few risks or side effects. Drowsiness is common, so someone should drive you to and from the dentist's office. A few people may experience hallucinations, nausea or vomiting. Injected sedatives carry the risk of small blood clots forming in the vein, which are merely painful if minor but can require anticoagulants ("blood thinners") and medical care if the clots are substantial and affect a larger portion of the vein.

Drug overdose is rare but is the most serious side effect. How, you ask, is this possible? Here's a possible scenario: The dentist prescribes premedication with a tranquilizer, uses nitrous oxide and injects a local anesthetic to carry out several procedures at one time. Miscalculation of the various doses can result in respiratory failure, cardiac arrest and death. Rarely, a kink in a hose or mix-up with the supply tanks may result in a patient receiving too little oxygen and too much nitrous oxide, with the potential for brain damage and death.

These remote but serious risks emphasize why you must not accept any sedation without question. Make sure the dentist has been properly trained to administer nitrous oxide, intravenous sedation or other sedative medications.

Ask how many people are involved with administering and monitoring the sedative. In addition to the dentist, at least one assistant should be present who is trained to monitor you while you are under conscious sedation. If the dentist is using nitrous oxide on you, a third person should be available in case you become agitated by hallucinations.

Most states regulate the use of nitrous oxide and issue permits. Ask to see your dentist's permit.

Ask about alternatives. Unless your fear prevents you from seeking needed treatment, local anesthesia should be adequate for most procedures. Several techniques are available to help you take control of your fear and anxiety, rather than simply masking it with sedatives.

WHEN IT'S AN EMERGENCY

Ideally, your visits to the dentist will be planned, involving preventive care or carrying out the recommendations of your treatment plan. In the real world, however, emergencies happen. Among the reasons to call your dentist for immediate care are the following:

- Injury to your mouth, teeth, gums or jaw
- Uncontrolled bleeding within your mouth
- Pain or inflammation that doesn't subside 48 hours after a root canal procedure
- Swelling and inflammation of the gums
- Tooth pain
- Broken or knocked-out tooth
- Broken or knocked-out bridge, crown or denture
- Missing filling
- Sores on your lips or inside your mouth that do not subside within a week

As we described in chapter 2, most general dentists have developed scheduling systems that allow them to see patients quickly in emergencies. In such cases, your visit to the dentist will be more focused than a preventive visit. The goal will be to correct the urgent condition, either temporarily, with additional appointments to complete the work, or permanently with one visit, depending on the extent of work required.

The structure of the visit, however, is much like that of a preventive one. History-taking centers on the circumstances surrounding the current condition: How long has it been present? What brought it on? What have you done to correct it? Have you taken any medications? The dentist carefully examines the area, gently probing. He may take limited x-rays to determine the extent of internal involvement or pinpoint the site of an infection. Despite the urgent nature of the visit, you should still be offered a treatment plan, probably verbally, in which your options are described. Despite your understandable desire to correct the problem immediately, take the time you need to ask any questions you have and to consider your options. If one option involves substantial time and/or money, consider applying a temporary solution if possible while you get a second opinion. Remember, too, that despite the fact that you consider your condition an emergency, your HMO or insurance company may take a different view. You may need to get prior approval for a costly procedure.

WHEN THE DENTIST MAKES A REFERRAL TO A SPECIALIST

As we emphasized in chapter 1, specialists play a much less significant role in dentistry than in medicine. Nevertheless, your general dentist may suggest a referral if (1) he has not been able to successfully diagnose your condition; (2) treatment is needed that your dentist is unable or unwilling to provide; or (3) you have a medical, physical or mental condition that makes dental treatment hazardous under general circumstances. You in turn may feel a referral is warranted if you disagree with the dentist about proposed treatment or if you have lost confidence in your general dentist.

Before you decide to see a specialist, ask the following questions:

1. Why should I see a specialist?

Ask your dentist to explain what he expects the specialist to do that he is unable or unwilling to do.

2. Why this kind of specialist?

You are looking for information about what this type of specialist knows that will be relevant to your case and what to expect this kind of specialist to do. Does the specialist only diagnose problems, or will he also provide treatment? If not, who will actually carry out the treatment? Would another type of specialist be preferable under the circumstances?

3. Why this particular specialist?

You hope the answer is, "Because she is the best in town." Bear in mind, though, that whatever the reason, with the relative scarcity of dental specialists, you may have few choices nearby. Many rural communities, however, are becoming part of electronic networks that allow distant specialists of all types to "examine" patients via videoconferencing to diagnose conditions and recommend treatments. You also probably have the choice of driving to a major metropolitan area and consulting with a specialist. If you know what type of specialist you need and you agree that the consultation is appropriate, don't let the shortage of local specialists convince you to accept less than you deserve.

Remember, too, that you do not have to accept the individual suggested by your dentist. If you are covered by an HMO, you can get the name of a participating specialist from your plan's member services representative. To locate a specialist, you can also follow the procedure outlined in chapter 1 for finding a dentist; details about training, certification and other factors to consider in choosing a specialist are also included in that chapter.

ON THE RECORD— YOUR DENTAL RECORD, THAT IS

Your dental record, like your medical history, is an invaluable resource for ensuring good dental care. It documents the care you have received, the dentist's notes, laboratory results, x-ray films, medications you've taken, questions you've had and communication between your dentist and your physician or dental specialists. A thorough, well-organized and accurate chart is essential documentation for both you and your dentist.

According to the ADA Principles of Ethics and Code of Professional Conduct, dentists are "obliged to safeguard the confidentiality of patient records....Upon request of a patient or another dental practitioner, dentists shall provide any information that will be beneficial for the future treatment of that patient."

Unfortunately, your dentist may not interpret that obligation as requiring him to provide you with a copy of your dental record. He may argue that you won't understand his notes, which could mislead you in decisions about care. He may argue that the records are legally his (which they are) and that once he releases a copy to you, he can no longer guarantee their confidentiality.

Whatever his objections are, you may be legally entitled to a copy of your records—depending on the state in which you reside. There is considerable variation among state statutes relating to access to medical/ dental records. Some states allow only patients' attorneys or health care providers—not consumers themselves—to have access. Other state laws refer to physicians and medical records, but do not mention dentists and their records, leaving applicability open to interpretation by state courts or regulators. We provide a list of those states with laws that give consumers access to their medical records (see below).

What can you do to maintain an accurate record?

- Start with your dentist. Ask for a copy of your record (you may have to pay a copying fee). Even if access laws aren't on the books in your state, your dentist can share your records with you. A good dentist should want you to be well informed and able to participate fully in your care.

States With Laws That Give Patients Access to Medical Records*

Some state laws specifically include dental records; others refer only to records of "health care providers." Call your state department of health for clarification of coverage in your state.

Alaska	Louisiana	Oklahoma
Arkansas	Maryland	South Carolina
California	Michigan	South Dakota
Colorado	Minnesota	Virginia
Connecticut	Montana	Washington
Florida	Nevada	West Virginia
Georgia	New Hampshire	Wisconsin
Hawaii	New Jersey	
Indiana	New York	

*Records in the following states may be available under special circumstances: Illinois, Maine, Massachusetts, Oregon, Texas and Utah.

Adapted from *Medical Records: Getting Yours,* by the Public Citizen Health Research Group, 1600 20th St., N.W., Washington, DC 20009; 202-588-1000.

■ Keep your own record, sort of a dental diary. Record dental visits, procedures carried out and who performed them, medications (prescription or over-the-counter) taken, allergies or other problems that arose during or after your visit and how they were resolved. Make notes during the visit or immediately after, while the information is still fresh. Be sure to note any recommendations made by the dentist.

■ Keep copies of all correspondence with your dentist, dental managed care plan or insurance company, along with a copy of your dental benefits handbook and insurance policy. This will help you monitor coverage, anticipate uncovered expenses and appeal if your plan denies coverage for needed care (see chapter 8).

■ Take your dental records along when you travel, especially if you received care just before departure, if you are undergoing a prolonged dental procedure such as orthodontics or if you have a dental condition brought on by a chronic health problem such as gum disease resulting from antiseizure medication. If you need emergency dental care during your trip, you can avoid unnecessary x-rays, medication interactions or inappropriate care by having an accurate, up-to-date record immediately available.

Your dental records are a valuable tool in retaining control over your care. Once set up, these records require very little effort to maintain, yet can reap substantial rewards to ensure quality dental care.

4

When You Need Treatment

I f you've carefully chosen your dentist and you visit regularly for examinations and professional cleanings, as we've described in the preceding chapter, then you may seldom need treatment for dental disease. Nevertheless, it is almost inevitable that a crevice will develop a cavity, a tooth will be chipped in a fall or another condition will arise that sends you to the dentist for more than a cleaning.

During these visits, you will want to continue the role that you established during your get-acquainted visits—that of an active partner. Ask questions, make deliberate and informed decisions and seek additional information and, if necessary, second opinions. Familiarizing yourself with your mouth's anatomy and related terminology is useful preparation for a dental visit. That way, you and your dentist can begin to speak a common language. You are better able to accurately describe where problems are occurring and to understand your dentist's recommendations.

ANATOMY OF A MOUTH

Your teeth are more complex than they appear. Whether they are the large back teeth, called molars, or the narrow pointed canines in front, all teeth are made up of four substances. Running vertically through the center is pulp tissue, which includes nerves, tiny blood vessels and connective tissue. The nerves and blood vessels connect to larger nerves and vessels through a hole in the root. As long as the pulp remains healthy, nutrients flow into the tooth, and the tooth remains a living thing.

The Types of Teeth

When you studied the human body in biology or health class, you probably learned the names of your teeth. Well, here's a quick refresher course. Now, when the dentist says, "That molar needs a crown," you can concentrate on evaluating the need, not on trying to figure out which tooth she means.

A full set of adult teeth is comprised of 32 permanent teeth, an upper and lower set of 16 each. Take a look in a mirror. Put your tongue against the upper center four teeth. These are incisors. Move to the left or right and you touch a pointed tooth called a canine (also known as a lateral incisor). Slide your tongue to the adjacent two teeth. These are premolars or bicuspids. The next two teeth are molars; if your wisdom teeth have erupted, you'll find a third molar as well. The names and relative positions are the same for your lower set of teeth.

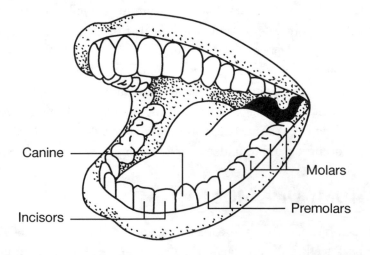

Anatomy of a Tooth

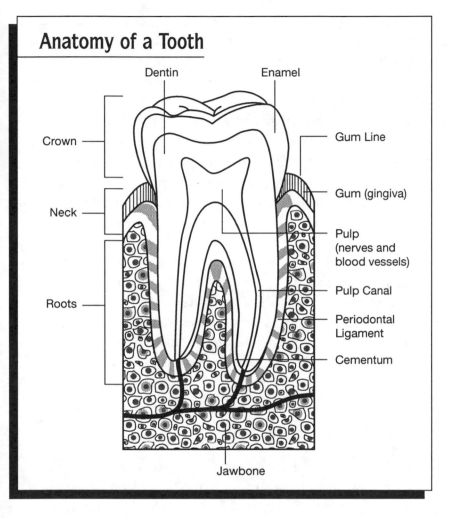

Dentin

Enamel

Crown

Neck

Roots

Gum Line

Gum (gingiva)

Pulp
(nerves and
blood vessels)

Pulp Canal

Periodontal
Ligament

Cementum

Jawbone

Surrounding the pulp and making up about 75 percent of the tooth's bulk is dentin. This hardened tissue contains living cells that are sensitive to temperature changes and touch when exposed. As long as nutrients flow through the pulp, dentin continues to grow throughout life, helping to protect the pulp when the tooth's outer layers are worn away or damaged by decay.

The outer layer of the root is called cementum. It is a thin, bone-like layer. Connective fibers, called the periodontal ligament, attached to the cementum also attach to the alveolar bone, the portion of the jaw that forms the tooth sockets. Like dentin, cementum continues to grow slowly, pushing teeth up as they wear down over time.

The portion of the tooth visible above the gum line, known as the crown, is covered with enamel. This is the hardest substance in your body. Lacking nerve endings, it is insensitive to pain. The thickness of enamel varies, with about one-sixteenth of an inch on the biting surfaces and one-forty-eighth of an inch on the sides. Despite its hardness, enamel can be worn away over time, especially in people who have the habit of grinding their teeth together. When the enamel is lost, the exposed dentin is sensitive to temperature and touch, causing discomfort.

When you look in your mouth, you see not only teeth but also several kinds of pink tissue. All of this lining tissue is called mucosa. Although it may all look pretty much the same, there are actually three types of mucosa in your mouth. One type, masticatory mucosa, covers the front two-thirds of the roof of your mouth (hard palate) and the gingiva (commonly called the gums). The second type, known as lining mucosa, covers the inner surfaces of your lips and cheeks, the floor of your mouth and under the tongue and the back portion of the roof of your mouth, called the soft palate. The upper surface of your tongue is covered with a third type of mucosa, what dentists call specialized mucosa.

A Name for Every Surface

In the language of dentistry, every tooth has five surfaces—and each surface has a name. You'll find these most useful when you look at your bill—fillings are billed by the surface, not by the tooth. So, for example, you might get a bill for three fillings but find them all on the same tooth. In fact, to your eye, it's just one large filling. The surface names are:

- *Occlusal* (the biting or chewing surface)
- *Mesial* (the side toward the center of the row of teeth)
- *Distal* (the side away from the center of the row of teeth)
- *Facial* (the side toward your cheek)
- *Lingual* (the side toward your tongue)

CONDITIONS THAT MIGHT NEED TREATMENT

As with the other parts of your body, your mouth is subject to illness and injury. Among the conditions are:

■ *Infections of the gums, lips and mouth.* Various bacteria and viruses live in your mouth at all times, kept from causing illness by your healthy immune system and good oral hygiene. These organisms, however, always have the potential to cause infections and may do so when your immune system is weakened, by a cold, for example. Among the common oral infections are cold sores, caused by the herpes simplex virus; trench mouth, a bacterial infection of the gums common among young people under stress; and thrush, a fungal infection involving all of the mouth's mucosa. Mild cases of these infections will usually clear up within a few days when your immune system is healthy again. Infections that don't improve in a week or that involve substantial bleeding, inflammation or pain should be seen by a dentist, who may prescribe antibiotics to eliminate them.

■ *Periodontal disease.* Also called periodontitis, periodontal disease is an inflammation of the gingiva caused by bacteria and plaque accumulating in the crevices where the teeth meet the gums. Mild periodontal disease, called gingivitis, is confined to the tissue closest to the gum surface and can be eliminated with careful brushing and flossing. If bacteria and plaque continue to accumulate, serious damage to the alveolar bone, gum tissue, periodontal ligament and tooth root can occur. As we describe in chapter 6, surgery to remove or repair the damaged tissue may be necessary.

■ *Tumors of the gums, tongue and bone.* Most growths in the mouth are benign. That is, they are not cancerous or life-threatening, unless they grow large enough to interfere with breathing. In fact, most may be little more than annoyances. Some growths develop as a result of a gap between teeth or irritation from ill-fitting dentures that causes injury to the cheek lining. Others may result from using smokeless tobacco, chewing tobacco or smoking.

Only about 7 percent of cancerous tumors occur in the mouth. The cause is unknown, although smoking, excessive sunlight, excessive alcohol consumption and irritation from jagged teeth or ill-fitting dentures seem to contribute to the disease's development.

Growths that don't disappear in a couple of weeks, that suddenly enlarge or change color or that interfere with eating or talking should be examined by a dentist. Benign growths can be removed by an oral surgeon and seldom recur. Small suspicious or malignant growths are removed by an oral surgeon and sent to an oral pathologist for microscopic examination and recommendations for follow-up care. For larger growths, an oral surgeon may surgically remove a tissue sample—in a procedure called a biopsy—for testing, and perform a second surgical procedure or prescribe radiation therapy or chemotherapy to remove the growth once a diagnosis has been confirmed.

■ *Tooth decay.* Decay of tooth structure, above or below the gum line, is caused by acid produced by bacteria as the organisms digest sugars remaining on your teeth after you eat. These bacteria, the most common of which is *Streptococcus mutans,* are found in plaque in nearly everyone's mouth.

The activity of the decay-causing bacteria causes calcium, phosphorus and fluoride (minerals naturally occurring in tooth enamel) to leave the enamel, a process known as demineralization. At the same time, remineralization occurs, returning these minerals from saliva to the enamel. If this process is in balance, teeth remain decay-free. But if bacterial activity increases or saliva production decreases, demineralization happens faster than remineralization, and decay results.

Some people are more susceptible to damage from the bacteria than others are, although the reasons are not always clear. A healthy immune system can keep the bacteria under control in some people. Eliminating the bacteria's food source by careful brushing and flossing after meals also helps. A professional cleaning, as we described in chapter 3, removes the plaque that harbors the bacteria, at least temporarily.

Decay starts on the surface of the tooth. If the bacteria are unchecked, the acid continues to dissolve the various layers down to the pulp. The extent of damage is a major determining factor in the type of therapy the dentist recommends to restore the tooth to health and function. Let's examine the common ways your dentist carries out this process of restoration.

THE COMMON SENSE OF COMMON PROCEDURES FOR TOOTH REPAIR

The Types of Fillings

Whatever technological developments have taken place in dentistry, one basic procedure remains essentially unchanged: When decay attacks a tooth, the defect must be removed and the resulting hole filled.

Millions of fillings are performed each year. Several substances are currently in use as filling material—amalgam, gold, composite resin and porcelain. The choice depends on the location of the tooth, the size of the cavity, the time available and your budget.

AMALGAM. A metal alloy that most patients call silver, amalgam has been in use for nearly 200 years. In 1993, dentists used an estimated 75 tons of the alloy, currently composed of silver, tin, copper, indium, palladium and zinc. Just before placement, the alloy is mixed with mercury.

Amalgam's endurance and popularity are the result of its inherent qualities. It is stronger than the natural tooth, is the least expensive of currently available materials and is easy to use. Within one appointment, your dentist can remove the decay and place the amalgam in a tooth. Amalgam is very durable, especially in small cavities. Studies have found small amalgam fillings intact and functioning after 14 years in 87 percent of patients and after 17 years in 78 percent.

On the other hand, its brittleness and need for support from the surrounding tooth make it unsuitable for large cavities. Its silver metallic appearance makes it unacceptable to most patients for filling front teeth.

GOLD. As a filling material, gold shares many of the better qualities of amalgam. Available for nearly a century to restore teeth, gold is very strong and durable and not brittle like amalgam. However, two appointments are needed to place a gold filling. An impression of the cavity must be made at the first appointment. After a laboratory has made a mold from the impression and cast the gold, the filling is cemented in place at the second appointment. Gold fillings take considerable skill to get an accurate fit. The additional time and expertise, along with the metal's high cost, make this an expensive alternative. Nevertheless, for

Should You Be Concerned About Mercury?

About 20 years ago, researchers showed that dental amalgam—metal alloy that is mixed with mercury to form the most common substance for filling material—released very small amounts of mercury vapor from a filling's surface. Since then, the American Dental Association (ADA), the U.S. Public Health Service, the National Institute of Dental Research and others have sought to establish if the levels released are sufficient to pose health risks such as the brain damage associated with consuming mercury-contaminated fish or the headaches commonly cited by critics of amalgam fillings.

We get mercury in our bodies from the food we eat, the air we breathe and other natural sources. These small amounts are removed from our bodies in our urine. According to the ADA, the average level of mercury found in the general public is 100 times lower than the level shown to affect health.

In 1991, the Food and Drug Administration and the National Institutes of Health asked panels of experts to evaluate the existing research on potentially harmful effects of dental mercury. These panels found no evidence that mercury in amalgam causes health problems. In 1993, the U.S. Public Health Service also reviewed the research data and again found no evidence that exposure to dental mercury poses a significant health risk. A 1995 study in the *Journal of the American Dental Association* reported no differences in test scores on mental competency tests between a group of elderly women with few if any fillings and those with many fillings. Less than 1 percent of patients receiving amalgam fillings may develop a skin rash as a temporary allergic reaction to the mercury in fillings.

Some dentists—and consumers—remain unconvinced. About 6 percent of dentists do not use amalgam filling material. Others will replace amalgam with other materials if their patients request it.   *continued*

If you have concerns, discuss them with your current dentist. If you need a filling, she may be able to recommend alternative materials. A few dentists recommend removing all amalgam fillings and replacing them, but you must weigh what risk you believe exists from the mercury with the potential risks from less durable alternatives and from the extensive dental work needed if you have many fillings.

For information on alternatives to amalgam filling and how to find dentists who offer such alternatives, contact:

Environmental Dental Association
P.O. Box 2184
Rancho Santa Fe, CA 92067
800-388-8124

large cavities with little remaining tooth, gold is the best alternative without replacing the tooth with a crown (see page 125).

COMPOSITE RESIN. The search for a material close to natural tooth color has resulted in composite resin (plastic) fillings and porcelain. Composite resin fillings involve mixing plastic resin and finely ground glasslike particles; this mixture is applied in thin layers with a bonding agent. The initial bond is quite strong, the color is often a good match with natural teeth, and a filling can be done in a single appointment. Composite resin fillings, however, can cause sensitivity if they come into contact with dentin or pulp, so a liner must be put into place before the composite resin is inserted. Over time, composite resin fillings can become stained, and gaps tend to open between the edge of the filling and the tooth. This allows bacteria to enter and decay to resume. At this point, the filling must be replaced. Composite resin fillings also require considerable skill to place them exactly so that they will last as long as possible. They wear away with abrasion from other teeth. This is not a factor if the cavity is on the outer surface of a front tooth, but it can mean a shortened life span for composite resin fillings in molars.

PORCELAIN. This is a ceramic material that is molded in a cast of the cavity and baked before being cemented in place. Longer-lasting and less subject to wear than composite resin, porcelain looks like tooth enamel, resists staining and forms a tight boundary with the remaining tooth. It is, however, brittle and difficult to apply and, like gold, requires two office visits to complete a filling.

Choosing a Filling and Having It Placed

Typically, in placing a filling, the dentist will first numb the area with an injection of local anesthetic such as lidocaine. Then using the high-speed drill with various sharp-pointed heads, the dentist removes the decay and prepares the hole for the filling material. If she's using amalgam or composite resin, she inserts the material firmly into the hole, runs a handheld steel explorer over the surface to identify irregularities and uses her handpiece with files and burnishers to contour and smooth the filling.

If you've chosen gold or porcelain as filling material, once the hole is prepared as above, the dentist inserts a short tray filled with impression material over the hole and the adjoining teeth. This is sent to a dental laboratory, where a mold is made and used to cast the gold or porcelain to the exact dimensions of the hole in your tooth. At the second appointment, the dentist applies dental adhesive to the cast filling and inserts it. She removes any excess adhesive, smooths the surface and burnishes the filling with the handpiece and her handheld instruments.

Only 2 percent of American adults will never have a cavity, so the chances are high that you will need to discuss the pros and cons of fillings with your dentist. Before you agree to have a filling, make sure you have satisfactory answers to your questions, including:

1. Is there any alternative to this filling?

If the decay is slight and has affected only the enamel, it may be possible to have the tooth treated with fluoride and return in three months to see if the remineralization process has restored the enamel at the decayed spot. If the decay is between two teeth, where remineralization is unlikely to be successful, or the decay is through the enamel to the dentin, a filling may be the only option. If the decay progresses to the pulp, infection and "death" of the pulp can occur. In this scenario, the treatment needs to be more extensive—and expensive.

2. Why is the particular filling material recommended?

The criteria for selection include aesthetics (or "the look"), durability, strength, expertise needed to carry out the procedure and cost. Your dentist should explain how the recommended material meets each of these. For example, if the cavity is small and located on the top of your molar, amalgam offers strength, can last 15 or more years, can be quickly and easily carried out and is the least expensive choice. It is not aesthetically pleasing, but few people besides you will ever see it. Composite resin would be more attractive but wears away on biting surfaces, may cost two to three times as much as amalgam and requires skill to place accurately. Appearance may be crucial to you, and you may be willing to undergo more frequent replacements to achieve a more natural appearance. Ultimately, it should be your decision as to which of the criteria are most important.

3. What are the short-term and long-term health risks?

Teeth filled with amalgam may crack after a number of years and, as we've noted, a few people (less than 1 percent) may develop a skin rash as an allergic reaction to the mercury in the amalgam. With all types of material, some people may have a sensitivity to temperature or pressure immediately after the procedure. This usually disappears within a short time. In a few patients, this sensitivity persists and requires a root canal procedure, which we describe on page 127.

Crowns for Your Teeth

Models and movie stars aren't the only ones who have their teeth capped. And aesthetic reasons such as a chipped tooth aren't the only reasons you might need a cap, also called a crown. This might be the best solution if you have a tooth with a loose or missing filling and too little tooth left to support a replacement filling; a large section broken off that may or may not be exposing the nerve; or extensive decay, the removal of which will leave very little tooth above the gum line. In each case, for a crown to last, the root must be firm within the socket.

Generally, the first step is to trim the existing tooth to form a miniature tooth or post onto which the crown will be attached. If too little tooth remains, the dentist or endodontist must first perform a root canal procedure, insert a metal post into the canal and build a miniature tooth around it. Then the dentist will make an impression of the tooth and surrounding teeth and gums, from which a model is made. This model is used to cast the crown, which is finally cemented into place.

Crowns, like fillings, can be made of various materials. Durability, strength and aesthetics are factors affecting the selection. Gold is the first choice for molars because it wears much like natural enamel and resists cracking, so it can last many years, even a lifetime. The most commonly used crown material is porcelain fused to metal. Tooth-colored porcelain is baked onto the surface of a metal crown. This provides a crown that is nearly indistinguishable from a natural tooth yet has a strong interior to resist cracking.

About 10 percent of women and 1 percent of men are sensitive to nickel, the major component of the metal crown. They risk gum inflammation and bone loss if a standard porcelain-fused-to-metal crown is inserted. People who have sensitivity to metal jewelry need to consider alternative crown materials, including a metal crown made primarily of semiprecious (palladium) or precious (gold) metals or an entirely ceramic crown. Ceramic crowns are a relatively new option, so their long-term qualities remain to be seen. They are, however, very lifelike in appearance, and because they contain no metal interior, they won't cause allergic reactions.

No matter what type of material is chosen, crowns are expensive—costing up to eight times more than a comparable filling—and require at least two appointments (more if a root canal is needed). Nevertheless, a good crown should last at least 10 years and many last 20 or more years.

A good fit, which results from a carefully made impression, is essential for durability. A poor fit may leave gaps between the crown and adjacent teeth for food to become entrapped and plaque to develop. The top of the crown must fit slightly under the gum without bulkiness that can cause irritation and inflammation.

When your dentist wants to "fit you for a crown," ask questions such as these:

1. Why is a crown the recommended procedure in this case?

2. What are my alternatives?

3. What kind of crown are you recommending? Why?

4. How much time will be needed?

5. What is the cost? How does this compare with the cost of the alternatives, if any?

6. What is likely to happen if we do nothing at this time?

A necessary component of your filling or crown treatment may be root canal therapy. Let's examine the circumstances under which you might undergo a root canal procedure and what to expect when you do.

Saving Teeth With Root Canal Therapy

Briefly, root canal, or endodontic, therapy involves drilling through the enamel and dentin to the pulp cavity, removing the pulp, ensuring that any infection is eliminated, filling the pulp cavity with an inert filling material and restoring the tooth with an amalgam filling or crown. With modern anesthesia and high-speed drills, it is a relatively painless procedure, despite its reputation.

The most common reasons for having it done are injury to the pulp from a blow to the tooth, a cracked tooth, deep decay or gum disease. Invading bacteria cause an infection, and eventually the nerve in the pulp degenerates and the pulp "dies," or becomes nonvital, in your dentist's terminology. If allowed to continue, this process starts to affect the bone and tissue surrounding the tooth. An abscess may form in which pus collects at the root tip and the bone will actually disappear. Without root canal therapy, a tooth with such damage must be extracted to relieve your symptoms and prevent further infection.

Symptoms that suggest you may need root canal therapy include the following:

■ Tooth pain that occurs when you drink a hot liquid but is immediately relieved by drinking a cold liquid. This particular sequence of "hot pain, cold relief" indicates that the nerve has been damaged beyond repair.

■ Sharp, acute pain when the tooth is tapped lightly with a hard object such as the handle of the dentist's mirror

- Discoloration (dark yellow, gray or black) on a front tooth or an un-filled back tooth. (Note that discoloration of back teeth that are filled with amalgam is common and doesn't require root canal therapy.)
- Tooth pain that is not relieved by aspirin
- Swelling of the jaw and/or gums
- Fever

The need for a root canal is confirmed by an x-ray. The dentist may see a dark spot at the end of the tooth's root or enlargement of the peri-odontal ligament that surrounds the root. When these are present along with one or more of the above symptoms, it is likely that the nerve has degenerated and you have two choices of therapy: root canal to save the tooth or tooth extraction.

Both general dentists and endodontists perform root canal therapy. As we discuss in greater detail in chapter 6, your dentist may suggest that a specialist do the work if you have a medical condition such as heart disease or diabetes that could complicate the procedure; you are taking medications such as immunosuppressive drugs after transplant surgery that could affect the outcome; or you have an infection that in-volves the bone. Endodontists not only can perform root canals, but also if necessary can cut into the gum and bone to remove a diseased root tip (in a procedure called an apicoectomy), can remove a diseased root entirely (root amputation) or can remove a diseased root and its crown (hemisection) from a multiroot tooth such as a molar. These pro-cedures, which are last resorts to saving a tooth, may be called for if the infection involves not only the pulp but also the root itself or the gum surrounding it. Large molars have three roots, and it is possible to re-move one that is diseased and leave two healthy ones.

Once the infected pulp tissue has been removed completely and the canal cleaned and dried, it is filled, usually with a natural rubberlike substance called gutta percha. Silver has also been used, but it has a much higher failure rate and should be avoided.

If an endodontist performs your root canal therapy, you will return to your general dentist for final restoration of the tooth. This can involve a simple amalgam or composite filling if the area of decay on the enamel and dentin is small. However, frequently these teeth have little crown left, either because of a substantial previous filling or because the decay affected a large portion of the tooth. In such cases, the dentist will have to install an artificial crown.

Root canal therapy is successful in 90 to 95 percent of patients—that is, the symptoms are eliminated and the tooth is saved. The more extensive procedures such as root amputation fail and require removing the tooth within five years in 40 percent of patients. The reasons for failure of a root canal are not always identifiable. The root may have tiny branches unseen on the x-ray that remain after therapy and continue to infect the area around the tooth. Also, the empty pulp cavity must be filled carefully. If you look at an x-ray taken immediately after the therapy, the gutta percha shows as a white line in the pulp cavity. This material should not show up outside the cavity or coming out the root tip. If it does, the dentist has put in too much filler. Nor should you see a dark outline of the cavity around the filler. If this shows up on the x-ray, the dentist has put in too little filler. Both circumstances often lead to failure.

If root canal therapy fails and symptoms remain (or return), the process can be repeated in some cases. Alternatively, an apicoectomy, root amputation or hemisection may be performed if heroic efforts are called for to save the tooth. Most commonly, the follow-up to failure is to remove the tooth.

The gutta percha can last a lifetime, but the outer filling or crown will wear and may eventually need to be replaced.

As you've probably gathered, root canal therapy can be time-consuming, which usually also translates as costly. While one appointment is possible, two visits are typical. Three visits may be needed if the tooth is a molar with two or more infected pulp cavities. It is essential that the canal be clean, dry and free of infection, which usually takes time to accomplish. If you need a post and crown to restore the tooth after root canal therapy, the cost can be nearly as much as removing the tooth and installing a fixed bridge (see chapter 6).

Some teeth are more important than others and saving them may be worth the time and money. Front teeth are the most obvious candidates for rescue. If you have lost several teeth in a row but have a remaining back molar, you may want to keep it so it can serve as an anchor for a fixed bridge to replace the missing teeth. If, however, you have all your own teeth and the problem is in a wisdom tooth, you may decide that having it extracted is the better course. Therefore, before you agree to root canal therapy, ask the following questions:

1. Why should this tooth be saved with root canal therapy?

2. What are the alternatives?

3. Will you perform the entire procedure? Or will you refer me to a specialist?

4. Will you use gutta percha filler? If not, why not?

5. What are the risks with the procedure?

6. How do you plan to restore the tooth? How long is such a restoration likely to remain intact?

7. What postprocedural problems should I anticipate? Pain? Temperature sensitivity?

8. Will the tooth require special care over the near-term or long-term?

9. How long will the entire process take?

10. What would happen if the tooth were removed?

11. How much will root canal therapy and restoration cost? How does this compare with the cost of removal?

Review the x-rays with your dentist. If, for example, the dentist wants to perform a root canal because the tooth is cracked, this is warranted only if the crack extends to the pulp. If you see that the decay extends into the actual root, the success rate for root canal therapy is much lower than when the decay has stopped in the pulp.

The proportion of American adults who have lost all of their teeth at any given age has dropped by nearly one-half since the early 1970s. In part, this is due to the use of the restorative services of fillings, crowns and root canals to save teeth that once might have been extracted. As with every medical and dental procedure, however, restorations can be overused. You can protect yourself and your pocketbook by remaining alert, asking questions, examining your x-rays and, if you have any doubts about a recommendation, getting a second opinion.

WHEN A TOOTH CAN'T BE SAVED

While it is true that Americans are keeping more teeth longer than did previous generations, circumstances still arise that require one or more teeth to be extracted. Among the potential reasons for tooth extraction are:

- To make space for misaligned teeth to be straightened by orthodontic work
- To eliminate a tooth that becomes reinfected after root canal therapy
- To prepare for partial or full dentures
- To remove a tooth that cannot be restored with a filling or crown because decay has destroyed too much tooth, the tooth is loose in the socket or another condition will affect either the tooth's longevity or the preparation of a filling or crown
- To remove an impacted (unerupted) tooth, usually a third molar (wisdom tooth), before it crowds the adjacent tooth or causes bone damage

Both general dentists and oral surgeons extract teeth. Oral surgeons are more likely to perform the procedure when the person has a medical condition such as diabetes that increases the likelihood of infections and other complications; the tooth to be extracted is actively infected; the patient must have general anesthesia or intravenous sedation; the tooth to be extracted lies close to the sinus cavity or facial nerves; the tooth is impacted and will require removal of tissue and bone to extract; or the tooth or surrounding bone structure is abnormal in shape or location, which calls for particularly sound anatomical knowledge and surgical dexterity.

Simple extractions are carried out after local anesthetic is injected near the extraction site. Once the anesthesia takes effect, extracting the tooth usually takes just a few minutes. A tooth that has broken at the gum line or breaks during extraction requires additional surgery to create a flap of gum tissue and remove a bit of bone to gain access to the root. After the tooth is extracted, the flap is sewn (sutured) into place.

Impacted teeth can offer the greatest challenges to the surgeon's skill, especially if the tooth lies on its side under the alveolar bone. To remove such a tooth, the surgeon must cut the gum tissue, create a flap,

The Wisdom of Extracting Wisdom Teeth

Old habits die hard. In the past, impacted third molars—wisdom teeth that have not erupted through the gum and bone—were commonly extracted in what was considered a preventive measure. Yet this procedure carries risks that have made many dentists question the wisdom of routinely extracting impacted molars. People undergoing extraction of their wisdom teeth are more likely to experience damage to their sinus membrane, leading to infection; damage to their facial nerves, resulting in paresthesia (see page 134); and stress on their facial muscles and jaw, leading to trismus (see page 134).

You may be the victim of unnecessary third molar extraction if:

■ You are between the ages of 16 and 25 and your dentist/surgeon recommends removal. Third molars are the last teeth to erupt, usually in your late teen or young adult years. Unless x-rays clearly show the tooth to be at a sharp angle that will prevent its eruption, take a wait-and-see approach.

■ The orthodontist routinely recommends extraction of wisdom teeth before applying braces to the other teeth in your mouth. While this may make his work easier by freeing up space in your mouth, even crooked impacted third molars often can be straightened as part of the orthodontic work.

■ One set of x-rays shows what appears to be an impacted third molar. Improperly angled x-rays can make teeth appear impacted. Make sure the dentist compares the current x-rays with your previous set. If you have no symptoms or discomfort from the "impacted" tooth, wait until your next set of x-rays to once again evaluate whether the tooth is actually impacted.

We have made this point before, but again, we urge you to get a second opinion before agreeing to undergo extraction of any tooth that has no evidence of disease or that has no symptoms, even a wisdom tooth.

remove the bone covering the tooth and then cut the tooth into smaller pieces to remove it. The flap is then sutured into place.

Immediately after the extraction, the dentist or surgeon puts a gauze pack in the space left by the tooth and has the person apply biting pressure. This allows a blood clot to form in the socket and usually controls the bleeding within 20 minutes (see question #2 below).

To state the obvious, having a tooth extracted is an irreversible step. While removing the tooth may eliminate one problem, such as pain, it introduces other potential problems. The space must be filled (unless the tooth removed was a third molar) with a bridge, partial denture or implant (see page 178). If it remains unfilled, adjacent or opposite teeth will shift, contributing to problems with chewing, pain and periodontal disease. So, before you agree to extraction, satisfy yourself that the benefit will outweigh potential complications. Among the questions to ask are:

1. What are the alternatives to extracting the tooth?

Tooth extraction should be reserved as a method of last resort. For example, even a tooth broken near the gum line can be crowned, rather than extracted, if the root remains firmly attached in its socket and is without decay. "Wait and see" is an alternative if the tooth isn't causing pain or bone or gum damage, as is the case in many impacted third molars.

2. What are the potential complications of the extraction?

Generally speaking, extraction is a safe procedure with few complications. For example, a study of simple extractions (without cutting into the gum) performed by oral surgeons found fewer than one in five patients experienced any complications. Most (85 percent) of these complications occurred during the procedure, involving a broken root that required cutting the gum, with no long-term effects.

Potential postoperative complications include:

- **Excessive pain or swelling.** Some pain and swelling are normal for one to three days after extraction. If they last longer or do not respond to aspirin or other nonprescription pain relievers, then you may have developed an infection.

- **Alveolar osteitis, commonly called dry socket.** This is an infection of the bone forming the tooth socket. The pain, which may radiate from the socket to the ear, doesn't respond to aspirin and may become severe.

■ *Osteomyelitis.* When the infection spreads from the tooth socket into the bone marrow, osteomyelitis develops. This infection causes deep pain, swelling, fever and weakness.

■ *Sinus infection.* This is a risk when upper teeth, especially molars, are extracted. If the sinus membrane is torn or punctured during the procedure, bacteria from the mouth enter and almost inevitably cause an infection quickly. Symptoms include a sense of fullness between the nose and ear, pain when the upper cheek is touched and a foul-smelling nasal discharge.

■ *Excessive bleeding.* As we've mentioned, for most people the bleeding stops within 20 minutes of the procedure. Once the patient is home, if the bleeding resumes, putting a teabag moistened with hot water over the wound and biting for 20 to 30 minutes should stop the bleeding (tannic acid in tea is a coagulant). If bleeding persists or resumes repeatedly, the dentist/surgeon needs to examine the wound and probably suture it closed.

■ *Trismus.* People having a lower third molar extracted or undergoing a prolonged dental procedure may have difficulty opening their mouth afterwards, a condition called trismus. Caused by overstretching and traumatizing the jaw muscles and joints, trismus usually disappears within a few days.

■ *Paresthesia.* People having a lower third molar extracted are also most likely to develop a lingering numbness of the lip, chin, cheek or tongue. Feeling much like local anesthesia that has only partially worn off, paresthesia is caused by injury to one of the facial nerves. It usually disappears within a few weeks but is permanent in about 1 percent of patients who have an impacted third molar extracted.

3. What type of anesthesia will be used and why?

We discussed the types and risks of anesthesia in detail in chapter 3. Here we want to remind you that whenever possible, local anesthetic injected near the extraction site is preferable to intravenous sedation or general anesthesia because it carries fewer potentially life-threatening complications. Furthermore, you remain conscious throughout the procedure, able to respond if the dentist puts too much pressure on your jaw (a cause of trismus and, rarely, a broken jaw). The cost is significantly less because the procedure can be done in the dentist's office without an anesthesiologist or other professional monitoring your condition. Recovery is swift, and you won't need someone to take you home after the procedure.

4. What, if anything, will need to be done about the space remaining after extraction?

If the tooth being extracted was a functioning tooth, not impacted below the gum line, then you will need to provide a substitute—a prosthesis—to continue the function. In chapter 6, we discuss the nonsurgical alternatives, including a bridge, which attaches an artificial tooth between two natural teeth; and a removable partial denture. Implants, artificial teeth that attach to a metal plate surgically implanted in your alveolar bone, are discussed in chapter 7.

While it was once true that losing teeth was a common consequence of aging, this is no longer the case. Improvements in oral hygiene, diet, access to preventive dental care and fluoride have combined to enable increasing numbers of Americans to retain their teeth. Furthermore, a conservative dentist who uses extraction as a last resort and a conscientious patient are a powerful team in avoiding extractions.

Although declining in numbers, extractions remain among the most common procedures in oral surgery. But they are not the only ones you or a loved one might face. We discuss other options later in the book. Before we move to the next chapter, however, let's briefly examine some of the other procedures calling for the skills of an oral surgeon.

UNDER THE ORAL SURGEON'S SCALPEL

You may need to consult an oral surgeon if you have any of the following conditions:

- Cleft palate, cleft lip and other birth defects of the mouth and jaw
- Benign or malignant oral tumors
- Fractured jaw
- Tissue and bone damage following radiation therapy for head and neck cancer or injury to the head and neck

- Misaligned jaws
- Temporomandibular joint pain

These conditions often require complex surgery to correct them and to assure proper functioning postoperatively. Surgery for birth defects and facial reconstruction usually involves a team of surgeons, including cosmetic surgeons, otolaryngologists (ear, nose and throat specialists) and oral surgeons.

These relatively complex procedures are performed under general anesthesia in a hospital or outpatient surgery center. As described in chapter 2, these settings must be carefully evaluated to lessen the risks of infections acquired during a stay, harm by incompetent or poorly trained staff, and unnecessary x-rays and other tests.

If you are considering oral surgery, take the time you need to get enough information to make a well-informed decision. Among the questions you want answered by the oral surgeon are:

1. What exactly does the procedure involve?

Make sure you understand which parts of your mouth and face are involved, where incisions will be made and what to expect in the way of temporary swelling, bruising, pain and restriction of diet or activities.

2. What result is expected?

Both you and the surgeon should have similar expectations to avoid postoperative disappointment.

3. How many times have you performed this procedure?

Crucial muscles and nerves lie within the tissues of your mouth and face; if they are damaged by an inexperienced surgeon, you could face a lifetime of pain or dysfunction. Someone has to be the surgeon's first patient, but not you.

4. What has been your success rate with this procedure?

Find out what complications the surgeon's patients have experienced, both short-term and long-term. Ask to speak with another patient who has undergone the procedure.

5. What alternatives to this procedure do I have?

If a tumor that is affecting your ability to chew or talk is being removed, you may not have an alternative if you want function restored.

On the other hand, if surgery is being recommended to correct jaw misalignment, you may want to consult an orthodontist to see if realigning your teeth with braces would give you a similar result.

6. What is the cost, and what is included?

If the procedure will be performed under general anesthesia in a hospital setting, you can expect to receive separate bills from the hospital, the anesthesiologist and each of the surgeons involved. During your evaluation visit, ask each practitioner about cost. Make sure you know who will perform follow-up examinations if more than one surgeon is involved and whether these visits are included in the fee estimate.

Unlike illnesses elsewhere in your body, problems in your mouth and jaw are rarely life-threatening. So you can take the time you need, get a second or even a third opinion and make a well-informed decision about treatment.

CHAPTER

5

Dentistry for Children

ifty-five percent of children between the ages of two and four have never visited a dentist, according to the findings of a U.S. Public Health Service survey. While experts disagree on just when the first dental visit should take place, they do agree that pre-schoolers who ignore the dentist altogether risk becoming part of the 42 percent of kindergartners with tooth decay.

The American Academy of Pediatric Dentistry recommends scheduling your child's first dental examination within the first year—that is, within six months of the appearance of your child's first tooth, which usually appears at about age six months. Your child's pediatrician can carry out this preliminary examination to identify any potential problems in tooth development or risk factors that could warrant an early dental visit. Such risk factors include the presence of a congenital defect such as cleft palate or developmental disability such as Down syndrome; residence in a community with nonfluoridated water (see page 146); and signs of tooth eruption abnormalities or areas of irregular enamel development (demineralization).

With or without risk factors, most experts suggest that the first dental visit take place before all 20 primary (baby) teeth have appeared,

Scheduling Your Child's Routine Care

The timing and type of dental care your child receives depend on several factors. Young children don't develop periodontitis (gum disease) or tartar buildup, so they don't need the kind of frequent cleaning adults need. If children practice good oral hygiene at home, their visits to the dentist can be farther apart than if they seldom brush. Here are some general guidelines to discuss with your dentist.

Examination

Age 12 months, to evaluate jaw, gums and other oral structures for normal development and signs of healthy tooth eruption

Ages 2-6, annually to check that primary teeth are erupting on schedule and without deformity or decay

Ages 6-14, annually to check that permanent teeth are erupting on schedule and without deformity or decay

Ages 14-18, annually or semiannually, depending on level of decay, child's oral hygiene and diet

X-rays

By age 5, one set of bitewing x-rays, especially if primary teeth are set so close together that the dentist can't visually inspect all surfaces

By age 16, a complete set of baseline x-rays of permanent teeth

Cleaning

Young children don't develop tartar, so the only cleaning they might need is for stains.

By ages 10-12, possible cleaning for tartar during annual examination visit

Ages 12-18, semiannual cleanings if tartar buildup occurs

which for most children means by the age of two. Among the potential benefits from an early visit are the following:

- Your child's first experiences with dentistry are pleasant, without the discomfort of fillings, crowns or extractions.

- The dentist can identify potential problems early and perhaps offer solutions that are less complex and costly than what will be needed later. For example, your child may be able to avoid costly orthodontics later by having a tooth removed during this early developmental stage.

- Your child can begin fluoride and sealant treatment before any decay is evident, at a time when these techniques have been shown to be most effective (see page 146).

- You and your child can size up the dentist in a calm, unhurried visit without the distractions associated with tooth pain or some other dental emergency. If you are unsatisfied with her answers to your questions or the way she interacts with you or your child, you can change dentists and not interrupt ongoing therapy.

- The dentist can answer your questions and demonstrate ways to head off decay or other problems.

PEDIATRIC DENTIST FOR PEDIATRIC PATIENTS?

Once you've decided to take your child to a dentist, the next decision is whether you need (or want) a pediatric dentist.

As we discussed in chapter 1, pediatric dentists have completed two years of specialty training after graduation from dental school. They restrict their practice entirely to children.

In a 1995 article in a special issue of the journal *Dental Clinics of North America,* David C. Johnsen, D.D.S., M.S., a pediatric dentist at Case Western Reserve University, described several practice trends that differentiate most pediatric dentists from general dentists when caring for children. First, pediatric dentists make different recommendations for therapy in some instances. For example, one study found that pediatric dentists were five times more likely than general dentists to recommend stainless steel crowns, rather than amalgam, for repairing a young child's decayed primary molars when evaluating the same case. While neither technique is right or wrong, stainless steel is less expensive.

Baby Those Baby Teeth

Your child's first teeth—called baby, deciduous or primary teeth—will eventually fall out to make room for the permanent teeth. But those primary teeth still need dental and home care. Here's why.

- Primary molars "hold space" for the permanent teeth. If one comes out before the permanent molar is ready to appear, nearby teeth can start to move into the empty gum space. Up to 30 percent of later orthodontic cases can be attributed to prematurely lost baby teeth.

- Cavities in primary teeth can cause pain or sensitivity to hot, cold or hard foods, which may affect your child's appetite and disposition.

- Infection from a decayed primary tooth can damage the permanent tooth growing underneath it.

- A prematurely lost tooth can affect speech and appearance.

The earlier that decay appears, the greater the need for treatment—and preventive measures. The primary incisors naturally fall out at about age five, the first molars at about eight or nine and the second molars at nine or 10. Cavities first discovered at these ages can probably be left alone because the tooth will make way for the permanent tooth before the decay can cause significant damage, but discuss this issue with your child's dentist should there be intervening factors in your child's case.

Because primary molars will be lost by age 10, the fact that amalgam lasts longer than steel is less important than in permanent teeth.

Pediatric dentists also recommend that children start visiting the dentist earlier than many general dentists recommend. General dentists often appear reluctant to care for children before age three or so, whereas pediatric dentists recommend a first visit be made by age two. In fact, a 1993 Gallup poll found that 44 percent of children receiving dental care under the age of two were cared for by pediatric dentists, while only 28 percent of children of all ages were. In part, this may be related to the special skills needed to manage this young age group, known to behavioral psychologists as "precooperative." Just getting such a young child to sit quietly while the dentist sticks her fingers in the child's mouth is a challenge many general dentists may not feel up to.

Another difference Johnsen points out is the willingness of most pediatric dentists to care for children with mental or medical illnesses or disabilities. A major portion of their specialty training deals with the effects of illness on dental disease and techniques for ensuring the child's cooperation and includes clinical time actually caring for these "medically compromised" children. Thus, pediatric dentists are likely not only to provide better care for this group of children, but also to be more comfortable in doing so.

With only children as patients, pediatric dentists have child-size equipment, child-friendly reception areas and, most important, child-friendly staff. As Ann Page Griffin and Jasper L. Lewis, Jr., D.D.S., M.S., noted in their article in the previously mentioned special issue of *Dental Clinics of North America:*

> It is impossible to overemphasize the importance of auxiliaries [hygienists and assistants] in the delivery of dental treatment to young children. Staff members must like and relate well to infants and children, understand youngsters' special fears and needs and be a source of empathetic comfort without being overly solicitous to young patients.

Of course, even general dentists can have child-friendly staffs and may have taken the time to develop their own knowledge and skill in working with children. Further, given that only about 2 percent of active dentists are pediatric specialists, your search for a dentist for your child may have to include more general dentists than specialists.

In chapter 1, we offered a number of suggestions for finding and evaluating dentists. These are applicable for your child's dentist as well—general or pediatric. Here are some additional considerations.

■ Look for an office in which at least one person is trained in Advanced Cardiac Life Support (ACLS), particularly the pediatric version. This training, offered under the auspices of the American Heart Association and the American Academy of Pediatrics, includes the proper use of cardiac monitors, oxygen administration and intravenous medications to stimulate the heart in an emergency. This is especially important if your child has asthma, drug allergies or other conditions involving his heart or lungs that could provoke an emergency during dental care.

■ Ask what percentage of the current patient load is children. The higher the percentage, the greater the likelihood that you've found a child-friendly practice.

■ Ask how the dentist gets his young patients to cooperate. As we discuss below, there is a range of behavior-management techniques ranging from distraction to physical restraint to medication. The child's level of understanding guides the selection of technique, but it is also true that many dentists, especially pediatric dentists, rely heavily on sedatives. For example, in a 1993 study of 2,000 general dentists and 1,000 pediatric dentists across the United States, researchers from the Medical College of Georgia found that nearly three times as many pediatric dentists (68 percent) as general dentists (23 percent) reported using oral sedatives on their young patients. Furthermore, 74 percent of pediatric dentists used nitrous oxide or other inhaled sedatives, while 48 percent of general dentists did.

A CHILD'S FIRST VISIT

Your child's first preventive visit should be a positive one for everyone involved. Let's see what one family's experience is.

Martha Jones and her son Robbie have chosen a spring morning shortly after Robbie's second birthday to visit the dentist. The reception area has a shelf of picture books, several boxes of puzzles and a glass-enclosed magnet game that catches Robbie's attention. He plays while Mrs. Jones completes his medical history form. Within a few minutes, the hygienist comes into the waiting area, introduces herself to Robbie and his mother and invites them inside.

Tips to Prepare Your Preschooler for the First Dental Visit

- Don't keep the visit a surprise. Your child needs time to prepare for the visit.
- Answer your child's questions honestly but without specifics. The dentist will be able to describe what will happen in appropriate terms.
- Don't describe your own visits to the dentist. A child's visit is usually different from an adult's.
- Play is one way children adapt to new experiences. Consider "playing dentist" with your child or a doll as the patient.
- Don't exaggerate the significance of the visit by promising rewards for good behavior.

The dentist introduces herself and suggests that Mrs. Jones stand behind and to one side of the dental chair, out of Robbie's direct line of sight. Mom will be able to observe everything, yet this gives the dentist the opportunity to begin to build a relationship directly with Robbie.

The dentist invites Robbie to sit in the special chair, a miniature version of the standard dental chair. She shows the child how the chair moves up and down and reclines. She shows him the dental mirror and the other examination instruments and answers Robbie's questions simply and clearly.

Before carrying out a complete examination of Robbie's mouth, gums and teeth, the dentist uses the "tell-show-do" technique so Robbie won't be unpleasantly surprised. First, the dentist tells Robbie what she plans to do. Using a doll, she then shows the youngster exactly what will happen and answers his questions. Finally, she asks Robbie to lie back and examines him. Throughout, she talks reassuringly to Robbie, verbally rewarding him for cooperating. She also asks Mrs. Jones a few questions about his diet and home dental care. When Mrs. Jones asks for suggestions to avoid struggles over brushing, the dentist invites

Robbie to sit on her lap and demonstrates, giving Robbie a new red-handled toothbrush to use at home.

The dentist and Mrs. Jones discuss the advisability of fluoride treatment, while the hygienist helps Robbie rinse. They agree to set a second appointment for a cleaning and fluoride gel treatment.

PROTECTING TEETH WITH FLUORIDE AND SEALANTS

Fluoride

Fluoride is a form of the naturally occurring element fluorine. Early in the 20th century, public health officials and researchers observed that some communities had much lower rates of tooth decay than others did. By 1945, naturally occurring fluoride in drinking water had been identified as the key factor, and optimum levels had been established. That year Grand Rapids, Michigan, became the first city in the world to supplement its water supply with sodium fluoride.

Today, an estimated 144 million Americans live in 10,000 communities with fluoridated water supplies or with significant natural fluoride in the water. Eight states and the District of Columbia require that some or all of their public water supplies be fluoridated—Minnesota, Illinois, Georgia, Michigan, Nebraska, Ohio, Connecticut and South Dakota. Alaska, Nevada and Massachusetts have laws that allow communities to choose fluoridation. While 90 percent of those living in the Midwest and having public water receive fluoride, only 20 percent of residents of Washington, Oregon and California do so. To find out the fluoride status of your water supply, ask your dentist, pediatrician or local public health department. If your water comes from a private well, ask the public health department about naturally occurring fluoride levels in your area and the availability of water testing services.

The American Dental Association points out that children who are born and raised in communities with fluoridated drinking water have had up to 65 percent fewer cavities than children living in nonfluoridated areas. Children appear to benefit most from fluoride because it is incorporated into the enamel of teeth as teeth are formed. This provides lifelong resistance to decay. In fact, a 1990 article in the *Journal of the American Dental Association* reported that compared with similar people living in a nearby naturally fluoridated community, 77 percent more adults who lived in a nonfluoridated community their entire life had teeth with evidence of decay in the root.

Fluoride also acts on the surface of teeth and thus can benefit both children and adults. Some research indicates that fluoride reduces plaque acid production that leads to decay. Fluoride also helps repair enamel during the earliest stages of decay.

Over the 50-year history of fluoridation, numerous studies have analyzed comparable communities with and without fluoride in their water supply. In a 1993 issue of *Journal of Public Health Dentistry,* Louis W. Ripa, D.D.S., M.S., of the department of children's dentistry at the State University of New York at Stony Brook, published a report prepared at the request of the Executive Council and the Oral Health Committee of the American Association of Public Health Dentistry. In it he analyzed more than 170 studies on fluoride, and with regard to risks he came to the following conclusions:

- Skeletal fluorosis, with symptoms of bone and joint pain and evidence of bone degeneration on x-ray, is found in individuals living in areas with high natural fluoride concentrations or working in the aluminum industry, where fluoride concentrations are high. However, no cases have been reported in the United States in areas where fluoride levels are 3.9 parts per million or less (fluoridated water is usually 1 part per million).

- Fluoride appears to act differently on different types of bone and so has both potentially positive and negative effects. Studies have found less osteoporosis and vertebral damage in women drinking water with about 4 parts per million fluoride compared with women drinking water with very low levels of fluoride. On the other hand, several studies have found a link between fluoride levels in water and the risk of hip fractures—the higher the fluoride level, the greater the risk of fracture.

- More than 50 studies of communities with and without fluoridated water have been carried out to establish a link to cancer, and several independent commissions have also reviewed available data. No credible evidence has been found that water fluoridation increases the risk of cancer. A 1989 study of sodium fluoride in rats and mice found an increased incidence of bone cancer in male rats consuming very high levels of sodium fluoride, but an earlier study found no such relationship. In 1990, the National Cancer Institute conducted its own study of human cancer incidence in fluoridated and nonfluoridated communities and, once again, no consistent link could be established.

- One negative effect has been identified—the occurrence of mottling or light brown staining on some children's teeth. Known as fluorosis, this condition is caused by taking too much fluoride internally. The teeth remain protected from decay, and the process stops once fluoride levels are decreased. Fluorosis doesn't occur when fluoride is applied to the surface of teeth.

For children living in nonfluoridated areas, supplements are available in liquid or tablet form to take during the years when permanent teeth are forming. The American Academy of Pediatrics revised its recommendations for supplements in 1995 because of increasing incidence of fluorosis and now suggests the following:

- Infants younger than six months should not receive supplements.
- Children ages six months to three years should receive them only if the youngsters live in communities with the lowest water fluoride content (less than 0.3 parts per million).
- Children ages three to 16 years should receive supplements if their water contains 0.6 or fewer parts per million.

Again, your dentist, pediatrician or local public health department should be able to tell you what the fluoride level in your public water supply is.

In addition to taking fluoride internally, children and adults can benefit from external (topical) fluoride. This is available for home use in toothpastes, mouth rinses and gels and at the dentist's office as fluoride solution or gel. Children who have had cavities at an early age, who have disabilities that make brushing difficult or whose diets are high in sugar or imbalanced from poor eating habits or illness are at high risk for multiple cavities. These children in particular can benefit from topical fluoride treatment in the dentist's office.

Sealants

Topical fluorides are especially effective in preventing cavities along the smooth vertical surfaces of teeth. Less protection, however, is provided on the biting or chewing surfaces. In fact, 84 percent of all cavities in children ages five to 17 occur in the pits and fissures of teeth, according to the National Dental Caries Prevalence Survey. Especially vulnerable are the large molars. If the dentist's fine probe tip catches within the pits and fissures of a molar's chewing surface, the risk of food becoming trapped and decay developing is high.

Sealants were created specifically for teeth with these pits and fissures. Sealants are plastic coatings that are brushed onto the chewing surfaces of molars. A study of Michigan children found that the odds of a nonsealed tooth developing a cavity were more than four times greater than for a sealed tooth over a five-year period. Furthermore, the benefit was even greater for molars that showed signs of very early decay (no visible enamel defects but a dark stain or chalky appearance, indicators of what dentists call "incipient caries"). When these teeth were sealed, thereby cutting off oxygen and food for the decay-causing bacteria, 10.8 percent of teeth developed cavities within five years. When left unsealed, however, these teeth had a decay rate of 51.8 percent.

As with fluoride, sealants are most effective when applied in children, just after permanent molars have appeared (ages seven to 12). Teenagers and college-age students, whose diets and dental habits are often less than ideal, can also benefit. There is less agreement, however, about the value of sealants on a young child's primary molars or an adult's teeth. Given the value of decay-free primary teeth, though, sealants may be appropriate if your preschooler is a high-risk candidate for decay, as described earlier.

In adults, traditional wisdom has argued that if a tooth has not developed decay by age 18, the chances are it never will. However, this doesn't take into account changing health status and habits. A number of medical conditions increase the likelihood of tooth decay, among them pregnancy, immune system disorders and an injury that affects the ability to brush and floss. Adults experiencing any of these circumstances could benefit from sealants on any molars that do not yet have fillings or crowns.

Sealant application is easy and painless for the patient, but the dentist must be careful to ensure adhesion. The teeth are cleaned, and the chewing surface is slightly etched (microscopically roughened) with dilute acid to help the sealant adhere. After the tooth surface is completely dried, the liquid plastic is brushed on. One type of sealant hardens by itself; another hardens when a fiberoptic ultraviolet light is briefly aimed on it. During subsequent dental examinations, the sealed teeth need to be checked for wear and the sealant replaced if it is damaged or worn down. Studies have found that up to 82 percent of the self-hardening sealants are in place after five years, with similar results for the newer light-hardened version.

If your child's dentist recommends fluoride treatment or sealants, be sure you know:

- The risk factors that led to the recommendation
- How long the treatment will take
- If parent-applied fluoride gel is an effective alternative
- The cost of the treatment and whether your insurance plan covers it
- The risks, if any, of delaying or refusing therapy and what, if anything, you and your child can do to lessen the risks

WHEN TREATMENT IS NEEDED

Behavior Management

A survey of dentists found that uncooperative children were among the most significant problems in their practices. No wonder. Dealing with a screaming, kicking four-year-old is exhausting for dentist, parent and child. Nearly one in four children seen by pediatric dentists has significant behavior problems. And almost every child may occasionally resort to whining, turning away or other uncooperative behavior to avoid treatment, manipulate the parent or dentist and attempt to cope with the situation.

The American Academy of Pediatric Dentists endorsed 10 behavior-management techniques for dentists working with children. The techniques, along with guidelines for their use, were published in 1992. Many of them parents may recognize. The 10 endorsed techniques are:

1. *Voice control,* changing your tone of voice to convey firmness (but not anger) to gain the child's attention and cooperation

2. *Tell-show-do,* telling the child what will be done, showing the procedure on a doll or model and then actually carrying it out

3. *Positive reinforcement,* using verbal praise when a child cooperates

4. *Distraction,* using video games, audiotapes and even continuous conversation to distract the child from the procedure to be done

5. *Nonverbal communication,* smiling, nodding when the child cooperates, frowning or shaking the head side to side when he doesn't

6. *Hand-over-mouth,* when a child fails to respond to other methods, placing a finger to the child's lips or the entire hand over his mouth with the comment that the hand will be removed as soon as the child quiets

7. *Physical restraint,* using a Papoose Board to wrap an infant during a procedure or holding an older child's arms to keep him from injury during a procedure

8. *Nitrous oxide sedation,* using a sedative given through a small breathing mask to relax the child but not put him to sleep

9. *Conscious sedation,* using a liquid sedative to relax the child but not put him to sleep

10. *General anesthesia,* putting a child to sleep so that major procedures can be completed without risk of movement and injury

As a parent, you know that getting your child to cooperate calls for different strategies, depending on the child's age, language skills, level of fear or stress and physical comfort level. Your own level of stress and fatigue and approach to behavior management also influence the outcome every time you want your child to behave in a certain way.

Your child's dentist will face similar challenges. In particular, John E. Nathan, D.D.S., M.Dent.Sc., of the Northwestern University Dental

School, points out that dentists who care for young children tend to adopt one of two attitudes in attempting to influence children's behavior. The authoritarian has high expectations for the child's cooperation and tends to shy away from using sedatives, but instead resorts to hand-over-mouth, voice control and physical restraint, if needed, to achieve cooperation. This type of dentist also prefers that the parent remain in the reception area.

On the other hand, dentists who adopt what Nathan calls the "child-advocate" style have lower expectations about cooperative behavior. Should a child become so uncooperative as to interfere with therapy, these dentists tend to resort to using sedatives.

"There is no objective data reporting which style is preferable," writes Nathan in *Dental Clinics of North America*.

Thus, it is important to have a frank discussion with your child's dentist before any procedure is carried out. Even though you may have discussed the dentist's behavior-management techniques during the selection process, the specific circumstances of an actual procedure may influence the dentist's choice of technique. For example, if your pre-schooler has several cavities in her front primary teeth, a sedative or even general anesthesia may be the preferred choice so that all the fillings can be completed in one visit.

Your dentist should bring up the subject of behavior management himself, but you must if he fails to do so. You should know what technique(s) will be used under what circumstances, exactly what is done and by whom and the alternatives. Remember: You can refuse consent to the use of any particular technique. Once a dental procedure has begun, you can stop the treatment up to the point that the tooth structure has been removed or a similar irreversible process has been begun. At that point, dental ethics require that the dentist complete the procedure.

You can insist on remaining with your child during treatment. (For more on your rights as a parent, see page 162.) The younger the child, the greater the likelihood that the dentist will suggest you remain. For some children, their parents' presence is reassuring and a positive influence on cooperation. For others, however, having mom or dad in the room incites whining, sulking and other misbehavior in order to manipulate the parent and avoid treatment.

A further consideration is your own fear of dentistry. Your child may sense it and respond, usually in an uncooperative way. If you cannot successfully overcome your fear, you may serve your child better by remaining in the reception area or at least out of the child's line of sight in the operatory.

Fortunately, many children today face fewer procedures and undergo improved dental techniques that speed treatment with less discomfort than did children 20 or more years ago. A positive childhood dental experience is a promising start to a lifelong acceptance of dental care.

Sedatives, Anesthesia and Pain Relief

No parent wants to see his child in pain or in fear. Yet before you agree to the use of sedatives or general anesthesia during your child's dental care, be fully informed about the risks and your alternatives.

"It is impossible to predict, with a reasonable degree of certainty, the clinical effect most sedative drugs used alone or in combination will have on a child, particularly a very young child," writes Stephen Wilson, D.M.D., M.A., Ph.D., and colleagues in a 1996 issue of *Pediatric Dentistry*. Unconsciousness, reduced breathing with lowered oxygen levels in the brain, nausea, vomiting and convulsions are potential consequences of the drugs used commonly in dentistry.

In the textbook *Risk and Outcome in Anesthesia,* University of Virginia anesthesiologists Frederic A. Berry, M.D., and Mark M. Harris, M.D., point out the seriousness of complications that can occur when an anesthetized child vomits and accidentally breathes in his stomach contents (known as acid-aspiration syndrome). This is a very rare event that occurs in about 0.065 percent of all surgical patients in the operating room and 0.033 percent of patients in the recovery room. One in five of the patients who develop complications from acid-aspiration syndrome either dies or is permanently brain-damaged.

Children also suffer a greater risk than adults of airway obstruction during anesthesia, write Lonnie K. Zeltzer, M.D., and associates in a 1989 article in *Pediatric Clinics of North America*. As Zeltzer explains, this is because a child's tongue is larger relative to her mouth than an adult's. When tongue and throat muscles relax during anesthesia, the tongue can fall against the palate and block the airway. The authors of

Smith's Anesthesia for Infants and Children note that such airway obstruction occurs frequently, with obstruction by the tongue as a major cause, along with preexisting nasal obstruction and spasms of the larynx.

In a 1995 issue of *Pediatric Dentistry,* Howard L. Needleman, D.M.D., and his colleagues from Harvard University reported the results of their study of one of the most common sedative combinations in dentistry for children: the sedatives chloral hydrate and nitrous oxide and the tranquilizer hydroxyzine. Examining the records of 336 young patients treated in the dentistry department at Boston's Children's Hospital, these researchers found:

- Sedation was effective in 81 percent of the boys and 65 percent of the girls.

Putting a Stop to Pain

Painless dentistry is desirable to both dentist and patient. Yet health care workers, including dentists, are stingy when it comes to using local anesthetics and analgesics (painkillers) with children undergoing procedures.

In a 1992 article in *Critical Care Clinics,* Judith E. Brill, M.D., of the departments of pediatrics and anesthesiology of the University of California, Los Angeles, went so far as to call the failure to provide pain relief "an unacceptable form of child abuse."

Other researchers have not used those words, but they do agree that children often are allowed to suffer pain in circumstances where adults would get relief. In a 1994 issue of *Pediatric Dentistry,* Peter Milgrom, D.D.S., and colleagues published the results of a survey of nearly 200 Seattle dentists. One in three of the dentists reported extracting or filling teeth without local anesthetic in some school-age children. One in three also never gave prescriptions for analgesics after tooth extractions. Finally, 10 percent denied that children even experienced pain with dental procedures.

continued

Why is surgery performed on children without anesthesia or their postoperative pain not even considered? Neil L. Schechter, M.D., director of developmental and behavioral pediatrics at Saint Francis Hospital in Hartford, Connecticut, suggests several reasons, among them:

- The incorrect yet widely held belief that children, especially infants, don't feel pain
- The belief by dentists and/or parents that pain builds character
- Difficulties in assessing the level of pain a child is experiencing
- Limited information on pain management, especially in children, in the dental school curriculum

So be prepared to be an advocate for your child by insisting on adequate pain control during and after dental procedures. Use the guidelines in this chapter to ensure that anesthetics and analgesics are safely and competently administered.

- Vomiting during the procedure occurred in 8 percent of cases, but did not result in serious complications.
- One in five children had at least one episode where their blood oxygen level fell temporarily below desirable levels, but it was quickly corrected by changing the position of the lower jaw.

Neither of these complications had serious aftereffects, but all could have. The American Academy of Pediatric Dentistry has issued guidelines to help ensure safe sedation for children. Among their recommendations are the following:

- The patient's blood pressure and pulse rate should be continuously monitored.
- The patient's blood oxygen level and ability to breathe should be continuously monitored.
- Only a licensed professional should give sedatives and tranquilizers (except for mild tranquilizers such as diazepam), and they should not be

given until the child has reached the office or hospital where the procedure will be performed.

■ Individuals carrying out the procedure should be trained and prepared to respond to any reasonably foreseeable complication.

Compliance with these guidelines usually means the presence of a dentist, pediatrician or oral surgeon to perform the procedure; a dentist, dental resident or anesthesiologist to monitor; and a dental assistant.

If, however, circumstances call for general anesthesia, then an anesthesiologist administers the drug(s) and performs some of the monitoring. Procedures requiring general anesthesia can safely be performed in either an ambulatory (outpatient) surgical center (see chapter 2) or a hospital. A child who has no medical problems beyond the condition needing dental care or anyone with mild medical problems such as low-grade asthma can usually undergo a major dental procedure in an ambulatory center, rather than in a hospital.

If you and your child's dentist have determined that general anesthesia is necessary—based on the extent of the procedure, your child's previous resistance level to dental care and his medical status—then you must evaluate the facility. See chapter 2 for more information.

Your more important task—and not an easy one—is to meet with the anesthesiologist in plenty of time to assess her capabilities and allow you to arrange for another one if you are dissatisfied. Traditionally, patients rarely choose anesthesiologists; the surgeons do, the hospital does, or it's the luck of the draw. Most people meet the anesthesiologist only the night before or morning of their operations. In your case, she will probably slip into your child's room, briefly introduce herself and start asking you questions about your child's health history. The idea is to find anything in your child's physical makeup that could conceivably cause trouble when he is anesthetized: allergies, asthma and so on.

Alternatively, especially in outpatient surgery, you may receive a telephone call from a nurse one to two weeks prior to surgery with a similar list of questions. You may not meet the anesthesiologist until just before your child is wheeled into the operating room.

That really is not enough. To be fair both to yourself and to the anesthesiologist, you should seek her out ahead of time. Ask the dentist who will be performing the surgery to tell you who the anesthesiologist will be. Ask for help in making an appointment with her. With that assistance, the tracking-down process becomes a bit easier. Anesthesiologists are independent vendors, so to speak. They sell their expertise to many hospitals; they don't have office hours (they may not even have formal offices). They are usually busy, elusive and tough to corner. But make the effort, even if you are able to visit with her for only 15 to 30 minutes.

- Ask many of the questions we've suggested for specialists in chapter 1 about her training, certification, experience and complication rates.

- Ask which kind of anesthesia will be used—general or local? Gas or injection? Why one and not the other? What dangers are there? (Even if your dentist has discussed this, it is a good idea to also ask the anesthesiologist. She has had special training and should be more knowledgeable about risks.)

- Ask if any preanesthesia sedatives are used with children to lessen their anxiety. (Lollipops containing a mild sedative are used in some centers; research has found that children who receive these lollipops are more quickly anesthetized and require less postoperative pain medication than do children who receive either no premedication or another oral sedative.)

- Ask about being present during anesthesia induction. Some hospitals encourage parents to be present during the induction of anesthesia, as their child is being "put to sleep," and in the recovery room when the child wakes up. Often, the anesthesiologist controls this procedure. (Be aware, however, that research from McGill University, Montreal, published in *AORN Journal* in 1988, found that parents who were very anxious before surgery became even more so after accompanying their children—and so did their children. Not everyone is up to the experience; you can help your child more by being realistic about yourself.)

- Ask if she will actually be present to give your child the anesthesia. Many anesthesiologists have such a large and geographically wide practice that they can't be at every operation they are responsible for. They hire help. In a teaching hospital, a resident physician, still in training, may be physically present. Or your hospital may use nurse anesthetists (nurses with advanced training in anesthesiology). Your child's anesthesiologist may merely check in by telephone from whatever other hospital she happens to be working in at the moment. An emergency situation could arise, one that only the anesthesiologist could handle, but she may be on the line to another hospital or too far away to make it in time. Insist that you want her physically in the operating room with your child, monitoring your child's progress in person. Accept no substitutes. Get it in writing.

- Ask about her fees. As independent vendors, anesthesiologists' charges are separate from the hospital bill. They are well paid, earning more than almost any other medical specialty. Check with your insurance company or managed care plan about coverage.

As with your child's other dentist and doctors, if during your discussion with the anesthesiologist something just doesn't seem quite "right" about her, arrange with your child's dentist or the hospital to have another, equally well-trained, equally experienced, board-certified anesthesiologist work during your child's surgery. And meet that person ahead of time.

Brace Yourself: Orthodontics

For many parents, dentistry for children means one thing—braces. The American Dental Association estimates that over half of children ages 12 to 17 have alignment problems serious enough to benefit from orthodontic therapy. About 4.4 million people, 80 to 85 percent of whom are younger than 20, currently are undergoing the treatment.

Orthodontics involves correcting deformities and irregularities not only of teeth, but also of jaws. If a person's lower jaw is larger than the upper, the teeth will not meet properly, a condition called malocclusion, and surgery may be required.

But it is the malocclusion caused by misaligned or crooked teeth that concerns most people who visit orthodontists. To correct this condition, a person may have to endure two or more years of bulky, sometimes unsightly braces (known as appliances to dentists); discomfort and often pain; a schedule that revolves around frequent orthodontic visits; abstinence from selected foods; and meticulous oral hygiene. Why would a parent choose all this for her child?

The predominant reason is for appearance and the effect it can have on a child's self-esteem. But crooked teeth can have other negative effects as well.

- Badly crooked teeth can contribute to speech defects. About 18 letter sounds in the English language involve teeth in making the sounds clearly and correctly.

- Crooked or crowded teeth can make brushing and flossing all surfaces difficult. This will give decay-causing bacteria a food supply and increase the chances of cavities and gum disease.

- When teeth are misaligned, they wear unevenly during chewing, and stress is put on facial muscles and the temporomandibular joint of the jaw. The result for some people is headache, facial pain, neckache, tooth pain and premature tooth loss.

- Some deformities such as protruding front teeth can result in mouth breathing, which dries the gum tissues and can cause them to become inflamed and sore.

- If the malocclusion results in teeth not meeting when biting or chewing, a person may have difficulty eating certain foods, a situation that can affect diet and overall nutrition.

The underlying principle guiding orthodontic therapy is to apply gentle, constant, gradual pressure to force teeth to move into better alignment. The oldest and most commonly used appliance for accomplishing this realignment is metal-band-and-wire braces. The modern version involves attaching bands onto anchor teeth at each end of the device, then bonding brackets onto the front of each tooth across which a wire is run from one banded anchor tooth to the other. Once entirely metal, the brackets are now also being made from transparent or tooth-colored plastic or ceramic, making them less visible than traditional all-metal braces.

The unsightliness of braces has led dentists to develop another option called invisible or lingual (tongue) braces. These are mounted on the back side of the patient's teeth and exert their moving force by pulling, not pushing, teeth into place.

Invisible braces sound too good to be true. For many people, unfortunately, they are. Despite their clear superiority in appearance, invisible braces have a number of drawbacks. First, because they pull, not push, teeth, they can't be used to correct all forms of malocclusion. Second, they are used primarily to straighten front teeth and can't be used if their placement prevents teeth from meeting. Also, they affect speaking and can irritate the tongue. These braces are difficult to install, require more frequent trips to the dentist for adjustment and repair and take longer to work than do traditional braces—all of which translate into higher costs.

You may also have heard of removable braces. These can be removed for meals or occasions when appearance is deemed "critical." The most familiar is the retainer, commonly used after standard orthodontic work to keep teeth in their new position until permanent stability has been achieved. Another type is called a palatal expander. This plastic plate fits into the roof of the mouth (palate) and gradually presses outward against the molars. It is used in young children to widen the upper jaw. Other forms of removable braces may be used to maintain space between two teeth when a primary tooth has been lost prematurely or to move the lower jaw forward.

Most removable braces are used in children. The forces the device exerts are not strong enough to change an adult's fully developed tooth or jaw position. These appliances are most commonly used before or after traditional braces, not as the sole form of treatment.

No matter what your age or the type of braces you ultimately need, your first orthodontic visits are diagnostic and designed to give you and the dentist the information you need to decide about therapy.

Getting braces is a major commitment in time, money and dental skill, so neither you nor the dentist should start without a solid base of information. Expect at least two and perhaps more diagnostic office visits before any work begins. The dentist will carry out some or all of the following:

- A full medical and dental history, including identifying any conditions that could interfere with your completing treatment
- A consultation with your physician and/or general dentist to discuss preexisting conditions
- An examination of your teeth, gums and jaw
- X-rays, especially a full side view of your entire skull (called a cephalometric view) with your mouth closed to demonstrate jaw alignment
- Measurements of your face
- Plaster casts of both jaws
- Color photographs of your face and mouth

As with all dental therapy, you should receive a comprehensive treatment plan on which to base your decisions about the therapy. You want answers to the following questions:

1. What condition(s) is the treatment designed to correct?

2. What treatment is recommended?

3. What appliances will be used?

4. Why is this particular therapy recommended?

5. Are there alternatives? How do they compare with the recommended therapy?

6. How long will the treatment take?

7. What result is expected? What are the chances of success? In the event of treatment failure, what results are likely?

8. What are the possible complications? Are there any potential long-term risks?

9. What are the effects, if any, of waiting six months or a year to begin? What happens if no treatment is given?

10. What is the cost? What does it cover? How is payment handled? Monthly? In installments?

Before agreeing to orthodontic treatment, you will probably want to get a second opinion. Also, check with your insurance company or managed care plan about what portion, if any, of the costs will be covered.

If your income is low and you live near a dental school, you may qualify for lower-cost braces through the school's dental clinic. Although more commonly providers of standard dental therapy such as fillings and crowns, university dental clinics may also offer some orthodontic care. Remember: As usual in a university clinic, you are a teaching tool, so you are more likely to be accepted for orthodontic therapy if you have unusual or challenging features to your case. The work will be done by resident dentists, who are licensed as general dentists and are completing their training in the orthodontic specialty. All work is supervised and reviewed by a practicing orthodontist. While the fee may be cut-rate, the dental care should not be. Make sure you have answers to the questions outlined earlier before agreeing to treatment.

PARENTS' RIGHTS, CHILDREN'S RIGHTS

Parents are responsible for ensuring adequate dental care for their children from infancy through their growing and maturing years—years when parents must make many decisions on behalf of their minor children. During the early years, issues largely revolve around working with dental care providers to receive competent, compassionate, safe care. You can and must exercise rights on behalf of your young child within the dental care system. With rare exceptions, courts have upheld parents' rights to make decisions about their children's care, under the presumption that parents are acting in the best interests of their children, unless their actions demonstrate otherwise.

A parent's rights are not total or absolute, however, and they become less so as a child grows older. State law and case law have defined a number of circumstances in which children under the age of majority (age 21 in Mississippi and Pennsylvania; 19 in Alabama and Nebraska; 18 elsewhere) can make medical and dental decisions for themselves.

But before we look at the major exceptions and at areas where children's rights may conflict with parents' rights, here is an overview of parents' rights.

With few exceptions, which we discuss later, parents have the right to make decisions for their minor children on the assumption that children "lack the maturity and judgment necessary for rational decision making," in the words of Robert Plotkin, writing in the *Journal of Pediatric Psychology*. Parents have a constitutional right to "control and custody" of their children based on the premise that they will act in their children's best interests.

A dentist, or any medical practitioner, is not legally permitted to care for a child without parental consent. There are two exceptions: (1) bona fide emergencies; and (2) several specific diseases or conditions, such as sexually transmitted diseases or pregnancy, where state or federal law permits a child to seek or approve treatment without necessarily requiring either parental knowledge or consent. (While this may seem irrelevant to dentistry, we describe just such a case on page 167.)

This almost absolute right of parents requires that dentists provide them with all the information they need to give informed consent for their child's treatment. Parents can give informed consent only if the proposed treatment or procedure has been explained to them thoroughly and all of their questions have been answered.

Parents have the legal right to be with their minor child at all times—in the dentist's office or hospital—and nothing can be done for or to that child without a parent's specific permission. This right to be with your child is essential for fully informed consent. Whenever it is necessary for you to obtain dental care for your child, you must be prepared to be assertive and, if necessary, disagreeable toward those who may attempt to deprive you of full participation in his care.

But there are some limits on your legal rights as a parent, as we've mentioned. There are certain circumstances or special situations in which the rights of parents may conflict with those of their child. In such cases, the interests of the child are considered separately from the interests or rights of the parent. As if that were not confusing enough, there are times when your child, legally, is not a child.

When Your Child Is Not a Child

EMANCIPATED MINORS. Historically, young people became emancipated—that is, they were considered self-reliant for legal purposes—either by reaching a defined age or through marriage or military service. However, in recent years, as Yale University law professor Angela Holder has pointed out in the *Journal of the American Medical Association,* courts have recognized the increasing independence of adolescents and granted them greater decision-making autonomy in a range of areas.

Among the legal criteria for emancipation, depending on state laws, are the following: (1) A teenager must be self-supporting; (2) a teenager manages his personal financial affairs; and (3) a teenager lives separately from his parents. Emancipation has been applied to college students, even if their parents are paying the bills, and to unmarried mothers. In some states, pregnant minors are also considered emancipated. In determining a teenager's status, courts have also taken into account issues such as the young person's responsibility for debts, ownership of property, tax status and parental disciplinary control. In several states, including Missouri and New York, courts have declared a minor emancipated who was still living at home but earning a living and paying room and board.

Emancipated minors can consent to dental care the same as can an adult. Holder and other legal experts emphasize that parental permission is not required, nor is notification of parents necessary. A dentist can take the young person's word about his independent status as long is it seems reasonable and sincere.

MATURE MINORS. Courts have also come to realize that teenagers who do not meet the criteria for emancipation may nevertheless be capable of informed consent for dental care. Generally, a "mature minor" is a teenager 14 to 18 years old, depending on state law or court decisions, for whom the following conditions apply: (1) The young person understands the risks and benefits of the proposed treatment well enough to give informed consent; (2) the care is for the patient's benefit, not someone else's (generally most relevant to medical transplant situations); (3) the care is necessary based on conservative dental judgment; and (4) the treatment is not a high-risk procedure.

When Rights Conflict

As a child matures, the potential for conflict between parents' and child's rights in the field of medicine is significant. Pregnancy and sexually transmitted diseases, for example, call forth the issue of patient (child) confidentiality. Marginally successful therapy for a life-threatening disease can bring about conflicts over the right to refuse therapy and the right to die.

Dentistry presents fewer, less dramatic episodes, but conflicts between parent and child can and do arise. Here is a review of some of the more prominent issues where child and parental rights often conflict.

THE RIGHT TO REFUSE TREATMENT. In competent adults, the right to refuse treatment, even lifesaving therapy, is generally upheld. The legal concept of informed consent requires that a dentist give a patient sufficient information to make an informed decision to accept or reject the recommended therapy.

The willingness of courts to allow parents to make similar choices for their children has been affected by a number of factors, including:

(1) the child's age; (2) consensus about treatment choices; (3) the effectiveness of the proposed therapy; (4) the life-or-death nature of the decision; and (5) the degree to which the child will lead a life worth living or of relative normalcy.

In general, in recent years courts have frequently been willing to intervene on a child's behalf against the parents' traditional rights in cases where parents do not appear to have the child's best interests in mind. These cases focus primarily on infants and very small children but also extend to older children whose parents have refused certain treatments on religious or philosophical grounds.

As a result, most doctors and dentists have become wary of these potential conflicts and, when disagreements arise, often seek to obtain court permission to treat a child without parental consent.

The situation is much less clear as a young patient reaches adolescence. John D. Lautos, M.D., and Steven H. Miles, M.D., writing in the *Journal of Adolescent Health Care,* point out that hospital ethics committees are involved in decisions to withhold treatment as often in adolescent cases as in newborn cases. Despite the frequency of ethical dilemmas with adolescent patients, no clear-cut or universally accepted guidelines exist for parents or dentists.

In their article, Lautos and Miles also state, "In theory, a mature minor, capable of consenting to treatment, has the right to refuse treatment. In fact, the legal doctrine on this matter is not at all clear."

Courts and dentists appear particularly willing to respect the rights of teenagers to refuse elective, rather than lifesaving, procedures even if the parents agree to the therapy. In one court case, for example, a 14-year-old refused to undergo corrective oral surgery for a cleft palate and harelip although his father would have consented. In a decision that was not unanimous, a court declared that neither it nor the father should force the boy to undergo the surgery. Holder goes one step further and argues that oral surgeons would undoubtedly refuse to perform purely cosmetic surgery on a teenager unless both parent and child agreed.

If you and your teenager disagree over her therapy in a nonemergency situation:

■ Allow time for both of you to get all the information you need. Do not be pressured into making a decision.

■ Make sure that both of you have enough accurate information to make an informed decision. For instance, your daughter may believe that scarring from the recommended surgery will be disfiguring, when in fact it will not; perhaps you could arrange for her to talk with another young person who has undergone the therapy. Invite a nurse, another oral surgeon or another professional that you and your daughter trust to answer your questions and discuss the options.

■ Look for areas of agreement or steps that could be taken that might lead either of you to change your mind: Can you both agree to abide by the recommendation of a second dentist? Or that you will wait for six months and then have the condition reevaluated? Aim for consensus, rather than confrontation.

As your child matures, conflicts in areas large and small, including dental care, are inevitable. If you have encouraged your child to be an informed dental consumer, not a victim, then you *and* her dentist must respect her decisions. Take comfort in the knowledge that you have armed her well to face off against those who would control her body.

EMERGENCIES. In an emergency, any child, no matter how young, can be treated without parental consent. Medical-legal expert Holder points out that under the law, an emergency is not restricted to a condition that may cause death or disability, but simply requires prompt treatment. In an article in *Emergency Medicine Clinics of North America,* Matthew M. Rich, M.D., J.D., chairman of the department of emergency medicine at Madigan Army Medical Center, explains further that legally, consent is implied in an emergency. Court definitions of an emergency have ranged from an immediate life-threatening event to situations in which pain and suffering are eliminated, for example, replacing a tooth that has been knocked out.

CONFIDENTIALITY. Whether you have a right to be notified that your teenager is seeking dental care or to know what is in his dental records varies considerably from state to state and with the reason for care. The simple fact that a law allows a teen to seek care does not mean that it guarantees confidentiality of that care. If the child qualifies as an eman-cipated minor, he is dealt with as an adult with regard to the confiden-tiality of the patient-dentist relationship.

Questions of confidentiality in adolescent dentistry are likely to involve sensitive medical information learned during dental therapy. For example, patterns of damage on a young girl's teeth might lead the dentist to suspect she has an eating disorder such as bulimia.

In another case, a 17-year-old girl, still living with her parents, consults an oral surgeon about removing her wisdom teeth. She and her mother consent to surgery. On the day of the procedure, however, when the mother is not present, the girl admits to the oral surgeon that she is probably pregnant. The surgery cannot be performed because of risk to the unborn child from the anesthesia. The surgeon does not tell the mother about the pregnancy but urges the girl to do so and to see a physician.

In cases such as the latter, reported in the *Journal of the American Dental Association,* "the courts have provided only limited guidance regarding the rights of adolescents to confidentiality," write the article's authors. "A general guideline is that minors who are allowed (by law) to self-consent for care should be afforded adult levels of confidentiality regardless of who is financially responsible for that care."

Nevertheless, each state tends to see parents' and children's rights a bit differently from another state, so the details vary widely relating to age, parental notification and authorized services. In other words, it is up to you to find out exactly how a particular issue of possible dispute is dealt with in your own state laws or how courts in your state have interpreted the laws. Call your family attorney, the bar association or a university law library in your state for more information.

Preparing for Maturity

Your child's maturation will one day lead him to seek dental care alone. You can do many things to help him and yourself prepare for that day. Begin during the child's preteen years. You and your child should discuss with the dentist issues of providing confidential care and under what general circumstances the dentist might feel compelled to break confidentiality. Encourage your child to spend at least part of an appointment alone with the dentist. Indicate your willingness to talk about what took place during the appointment, but don't insist that your child tell you anything or everything.

As your child reaches an age when he can make his own appointments and arrangements for transportation, discuss with him and the dentist how you want to handle paying for the care without jeopardizing confidentiality.

If you and your child have been going to a family or general practitioner, rather than a pediatric dentist, there is no reason that your child can't continue receiving care indefinitely from the same dentist if the relationship has been satisfactory. However, both you and the dentist must respect your maturing child's right to seek care from another dentist he feels more comfortable with. Pediatric dentists with knowledge and interest in adolescent care may continue to treat their young patients until they reach maturity and beyond. Again, it's really up to your child to decide; there is no magic date that signals when to move on to another practitioner.

In getting dental care for your child at any age, we urge you to ask questions, to seek alternatives, to be involved in your child's care and to involve your child in his own care. With this background, an adolescent is better prepared to use dental resources when they are needed and to evaluate his alternatives wisely. You have given him a solid start on the road to being an informed partner in caring for his lifelong dental health and well-being.

Dentistry for People With Special Needs

U p to now, we've covered procedures and issues that are likely to come up for anyone seeking quality dental care. But dental needs are not homogeneous; they change over time and are affected by existing physical and mental conditions such as pregnancy, diabetes or Alzheimer's disease. Older people and, in fact, *anyone* with illnesses and disabilities offer significant challenges to dentistry. The profession has a name for these patients—special needs patients. The dental curriculum assigns training time to their needs, and the profession even has a journal, *Special Care in Dentistry,* devoted to issues of their care.

All this professional attention is valuable, but it doesn't lessen the necessity for you to be informed and vigilant when seeking dental care for yourself or a loved one with special needs. You may face indifference, incompetence or reluctance when you look for care. Knowledge of some of the key issues will help you succeed in your role as dental advocate. We'll start with care for older people.

DENTAL CARE FOR THE ELDERLY

People ages 65 and older have been among the most visible groups of Americans benefitting significantly from dental advances during recent decades. More than 31 million people—12.5 percent of the population—were 65 or older at the 1990 census. Estimates are that one in seven Americans will be 65 or older in 2020.

Forty years ago, 60 percent of people in this age group had lost all their natural teeth. Not so today. The most recent National Survey of Oral Health, carried out in 1985-86 by the National Institute of Dental Research (NIDR), found that 41 percent of seniors no longer had any natural teeth. Of those in the youngest category of seniors, 65 to 69 years, fully two-thirds still had some or all of their teeth, while about half of those in their 80s did.

That is good news, indeed. Americans are keeping more teeth longer because of greater access to and improvements in dental care; the effects of fluoridation; improved oral hygiene; and changes in dental philosophy that encourage tooth restoration rather than extraction.

Nevertheless, aging still affects oral health. Kenneth Shay, D.D.S., M.S., of the University of Michigan School of Dentistry, points to the nearly universal prevalence of bone loss resulting from periodontitis (gum disease) in older patients. People who retain teeth continue to be susceptible to this bacterial disease; in fact, studies have found that periodontitis and related bone loss occur at an accelerated rate in older people. With bone loss comes loss of attachment of the tooth's root, which loosens the tooth and creates tiny spaces between root and gum where plaque accumulates. As a result, nearly three times as many older adults have root cavities as do younger working adults, according to the NIDR study. (There's more on periodontal disease and therapy later in this chapter.)

Retaining natural teeth also means that fillings and crowns that were put into place years earlier begin to fail and must be replaced. Even natural teeth without any restoration begin to show signs of wear. This wear causes temperature sensitivity and greater susceptibility to decay.

Aging also brings a greater risk of other oral diseases. In the United States, 90 percent of oral cancer cases occur in individuals age 50 or older. Cancer of the mouth and throat is the sixth most common cancer found in American men, especially in those who use tobacco or alcohol.

For most older people, aging also brings various medical conditions, some of them chronic, that can have a direct or indirect impact on oral health. For example, about one in 10 older adults have type 2 diabetes mellitus. This disease is associated with slow wound healing, a decreased ability to fight infection and increased incidence of periodontitis. As a result, any dental procedures that involve cutting into the gum and/or bone require special precautions.

Diseases that bring disability, such as arthritis and stroke, often bring dental concerns as well. Patients may be unable to brush and floss adequately, to travel easily for dental appointments or to sit in a standard dental chair. Patients with rheumatoid arthritis may be taking corticosteroids that can increase the risk of bacteremia (the presence of bacteria in the blood) after dental procedures. The medicines that stroke patients are likely to be taking to prevent blood clots could result in excessive bleeding after dental work.

In fact, medications can be a factor in dental health and care for nearly every elderly person in at least three other ways. First, an estimated four out of five elderly people have one or more chronic illnesses, and most take one or more medications to treat them. Shay notes that "an extremely common side effect of a vast number of both prescription and nonprescription medications" is dry mouth, known medically as xerostomia. This is a side effect of drugs given for urinary incontinence, depression, hypertension, dizziness, anxiety, pain and inflammation, among others. When saliva flow is reduced, oral bacteria and plaque increase, often resulting in periodontitis and tooth decay.

The second way that medications affect dental care is potential interaction between drugs already being taken for a medical condition and those newly prescribed for a dental one. And finally, older people are often more sensitive to the effects of medications, including those used in dentistry, than are younger patients.

Confronting Ageism

Thirty years ago, researchers coined the term *ageism* to describe negative attitudes or prejudices against a particular age group. The term now is generally applied to attitudes toward older people. Various studies of psychiatrists, health care workers and dentists have identified ageist attitudes that may prevent older patients from getting the care they need. Many older people, however, don't need researchers to tell them how stereotypes have affected their care. They experience them with every office visit or telephone call.

Among the incorrect beliefs commonly held by dentists, and even by older patients themselves and their families, that may influence dental therapy are the following:

- Older patients can't tolerate long or extensive dental procedures.
- Wounds in older patients don't heal well.
- The elderly can't afford major dental work.
- Losing teeth is an inevitable aspect of aging.
- A patient who no longer has any teeth has little need for regular dental care.
- Older patients are difficult to work with.
- An older patient's life expectancy doesn't justify extensive or expensive dental procedures.

Such beliefs can influence a dentist to offer fewer options to treat a problem, presenting only the less expensive or less extensive treatments. These stereotypical beliefs can be used to justify taking less time to evaluate and diagnose a condition. Combined with the fact that few practicing dentists have had any training in geriatrics, these misconceptions can result in needless complications from drug interactions, pain from untreated decay or other dental disease, and lower quality of life from less-than-satisfactory therapy.

WHEN TREATMENT IS NEEDED

Periodontal Disease

As we described in chapter 4, when plaque collects in the crevice where the tooth and gingiva meet, bacteria cause inflammation called gingivitis. This condition can be eliminated and prevented from recurring by a professional cleaning and careful brushing and flossing. When plaque continues to build, however, gingiva pulls away from the tooth. The tiny pocket formed signals the start of periodontitis. The deeper the pocket, the more serious the disease.

A National Institute of Dental Research study found that more than 95 percent of seniors have at least one pocket 2 millimeters or greater in

Ensuring Senior-Friendly Care

- Look for a dentist who has been in practice for several years and has treated other older patients. Research has found that dentists who have been practicing longer and those who have more experience caring for older patients hold fewer stereotypes.

- Look for outward signs of a "seniors welcome" practice— wheelchair-accessible office; firm reception area seating so seniors with joint problems can rise easily; forms in large print on nonglare paper; reading materials of interest to older patients; a well-lit office with no area rugs or step-up/down thresholds; transportation assistance to dental appointments, and so on.

- Look for a dentist who requests a detailed drug history, including regular updates at each visit.

- If visits for an examination and cleaning are shorter than they were a few years earlier (or with your previous dentist), ask why. Preventive measures are just as important now as when you were younger.

- When your dentist outlines a treatment plan, ask why he recommends the particular treatments. Are others available? Would he make a different recommendation if you were, say, 45 years old? Why?

- If you are being treated for a medical condition such as hypertension, rheumatoid arthritis or kidney failure, ask your doctor about precautions during dental therapy. Don't assume your dentist knows about the disease and its impact on his therapy. If you have printed materials on your condition, give a copy to the dentist. Encourage him to call your physician. Remind him about your illness and drugs you're taking before agreeing to any major treatment or accepting any dental medications. (For more on dentistry when you are ill, see page 187.)

depth—that is, signs of moderate periodontitis. Less than one-quarter had serious disease (at least one tooth with a pocket of 4 millimeters or greater). Researchers comparing these findings with results from earlier studies are optimistic that most of us face less serious gum disease than earlier generations did. Nevertheless, as more of us keep more teeth longer, we'll continue to be susceptible to periodontal disease.

Among the indications that you may have periodontal disease are frequent bleeding when you brush or floss, redness or slight swelling along the gum line, and loose teeth.

Depending on the severity of your periodontal disease, several levels of therapy are currently available.

SCALING AND ROOT PLANING. Using stainless steel scalers with a curved or hooked end, the dentist or hygienist first scrapes away the deposits of hardened plaque, called calculus. Then she planes the root to remove a very thin layer of the cementum, the outer shell of the root, providing a smooth surface for the gum to reattach to.

If the periodontitis has been caught early (shallow pockets, little or no bone loss), this procedure may be all that is needed to correct the condition. Regular professional cleaning (see chart on following page) and very thorough brushing and flossing can then keep the bacteria under control.

PERIODONTAL SURGERY OF GUMS. If pockets are very deep (6 millimeters or more) or if scaling and planing have failed to correct the periodontitis, you may be a candidate for gum surgery.

The most commonly performed procedure is called open-flap (or simply flap) surgery. The dentist cuts the gum tissue to the bone, leaving the lower edge attached. Pulling away this flap reveals the tooth's root(s) and allows for scraping and planing the entire root surface. The flap is put back into position and sewn with sutures, which are removed five to six days later.

In otherwise healthy patients, this type of gum surgery can be performed by a periodontist or oral surgeon in his office or an ambulatory surgery center (see chapter 2). There are few risks except for patients allergic to anesthesia (see chapter 3).

It is important to note, however, that various studies have shown that neither the nonsurgical nor the surgical procedures are cures for periodontal disease. Once it becomes evident, periodontitis is a chronic condition that may be eliminated in one tooth only to flare up in another. Keeping it under control may be the best many patients can expect.

PERIODONTAL SURGERY INVOLVING BONE. At one time, patients with advanced periodontal disease almost inevitably faced tooth loss and dentures. Modern dentistry, however, offers surgical procedures that encourage lost tissue to regenerate or use grafts to fill bone defects. One procedure, called guided tissue regeneration, involves carrying out flap surgery as described above, scraping and root planing, and covering the bone defect with a membrane that fits tightly against the tooth. The gum flap is sewn into place. After six weeks, the membrane is removed.

The Timing of Care

You may be able to avoid extensive periodontal surgery by getting regular gum care. Follow these guidelines to plan your dental visits.

CONDITION	POCKET DEPTH (MILLIMETERS)	VISIT FREQUENCY (MONTHS)	PROCEDURE(S) CARRIED OUT
Gingivitis & early periodontitis	4 or less	6-12	Exam; cleaning; scaling
Moderate periodontitis	4-6	3-4	Exam; root planing initially & as needed; cleaning; scaling
Advanced periodontitis	More than 6	3	Exam; scaling; root planing; periodontal surgery initially & as needed

Source: Adapted from *Complete Guide to Dental Health.* J.W. Friedman and the Editors of Consumer Reports Books. Yonkers, N.Y.: Consumer Reports Books, 1991.

Ligament and bone tissue have regrown to partially or completely fill the space.

In some patients, bone loss can be corrected by grafting new bone or bone substitute at the site of the defect. Once again, a flap is cut into the gum. The bone defect is filled with tiny particles of graft material and then the flap is reattached.

Three types of bone graft material are used in this periodontal surgery: autograft (patient's own bone), allograft (bone particles from a tissue bank) and alloplast (synthetic bone particles). As you can probably guess, these graft procedures are relatively complex surgical operations. Each type has distinct advantages and disadvantages, so be sure to thoroughly discuss the issue with your practitioner.

Periodontists and oral surgeons have been trained to carry out these procedures. In some communities, you may also find a general dentist who has undergone additional training to perform the graft regeneration technique and even graft surgery. No matter what title or specialty the dentist uses, you want to know:

1. How many similar procedures has she performed?

Experience and skill are essential to success. This is not the time to be first.

2. Why does she want to carry out this procedure in this case?

Both guided tissue regeneration and graft surgery are most successful in the lower jaw with holes in the bone that still retain their sides, rather than flat worn spots. Regeneration also performs well if the bone defect is immediately adjacent to a tooth root. If the dentist proposes surgery for your upper jaw or for bone with a less defined defect, ask what her success rate has been and why she believes you are still a candidate for the surgery.

3. What complications have her patients experienced?

4. How long is the recovery period likely to be?

5. What are the alternatives, if any, to surgery?

If she recommends an autograft, you want to know:

1. Why use an autograft rather than an allograft?

2. Where will she take the graft bone from?

3. How long will the two procedures take?

4. If it fails, can another type of graft be tried?

If she recommends an allograft, find out:

1. What is her source for the bone graft tissue?

2. Is the tissue bank accredited by the American Association of Tissue Banks?

3. Does the tissue bank routinely carry out HIV and DNA tests?

4. How did she select this particular bank? How long has she used it?

5. Have any of her patients developed complications such as infections that were traced to the bank?

6. What has been her success rate with allografts?

7. Why does she recommend an allograft over an autograft?

Given that current alloplast materials have a low success rate, few dentists outside a research center are likely to use them. However, as research continues, new and better materials may make this a successful alternative for individuals who cannot use their own bone and will not use cadaver bone. If your dentist recommends an alloplast graft, find out:

1. How long has this particular material been in general use? How long has she used it?

2. What has the success rate been with this particular material?

3. Why has she selected this particular material?

No matter what graft procedure you are considering, ask to see x-ray films of another patient before and several years after your dentist performed the same procedure. You should be able to see the bone defect as a dark spot on the "before" x-ray and none on the "after."

Get at least one other opinion. As we've said before, this is relatively complex surgery and should not be agreed to without as much information as possible. If you have a medical condition such as heart disease or diabetes, insist that your dentist and doctor discuss the advisability of the surgery and what precautions (if any) to take.

Ask also where the procedure will be done. Use the guidelines in chapter 2 to evaluate the location's acceptability.

Replacing Missing Teeth

As we noted at the beginning of this chapter, losing all your teeth is no longer an inevitable consequence of the aging process. Nearly everyone will have one or more artificial teeth by the age of 65.

These artificial teeth, in the form of crowns, bridges, dentures and implants, are the focus of prosthodontics. (See chapter 4 for more information on crowns and chapter 7 for a discussion of implants.)

Less than 2 percent of dentists specialize in prosthodontics. Most artificial teeth are placed by general dentists.

WHEN ONLY A FEW TEETH ARE MISSING. If you have lost only a few teeth—a couple of your back molars or no more than four front teeth— you may get a bridge. Three types are currently used: the standard fixed bridge, the cantilever bridge and the Maryland bridge.

To Replace or Not to Replace

When you lose a tooth, you have the option of not replacing it. This is especially tempting in the case of lost molars, which are not visible when you talk. However, before making that decision, look at what happens to your remaining teeth when a tooth is lost.

- Teeth adjacent to the space slide toward each other.
- Space opens between teeth adjacent to the missing tooth and the next teeth, creating places for food and bacteria to become trapped.
- The tooth opposite the space elongates.
- Resulting tooth misalignment can affect chewing and jaw alignment and put destructive stress on misaligned teeth.

The most common type is the fixed bridge, also among the most expensive treatments in general dentistry. The artificial tooth (porcelain or plastic/resin) is permanently attached to sound teeth on each side of the gap created by the missing tooth. The supporting teeth must be firmly set in their sockets to bear the weight of the artificial tooth. Typically, crowns are put on these supporting teeth to lessen the chance of decay.

If you have lost your front incisor, you may choose a special kind of fixed bridge called a cantilever bridge. Here the artificial tooth is attached on one side only, to the adjacent "canine" tooth.

The Maryland bridge—whose official name is resin-bonded fixed partial denture—is used to replace one or more teeth. As with the standard fixed bridge, the artificial tooth is attached to adjacent healthy teeth. The Maryland bridge, however, is designed so that less damage is done to those supporting teeth. For front tooth replacement, the back (lingual) side of the supporting teeth is etched to create a rough surface and shallow grooves. If a molar is being replaced, the chewing surface of adjoining molars is similarly etched. The artificial tooth has two "wings" made of a nickel-based alloy (or gold for those allergic to nickel), which are bonded to the supporting teeth with plastic cement (resin).

A removable partial denture is an alternative to these fixed bridges when only some of your teeth must be replaced. The artificial teeth, made of tooth-colored plastic, are mounted in pink plastic, which in turn is mounted onto a metal alloy (usually chrome-cobalt) framework. The horseshoe-shaped framework extends to the opposite side of the jaw and includes metal clasps that encircle remaining teeth. Physical support comes from the jawbone, gums and teeth.

A recent refinement in removable partial dentures has a similar structure, but instead of clasps, it uses precision attachments. Supporting teeth are fitted with crowns that have tiny vertical slots in them. The denture's framework has tabs precisely designed to fit these slots, holding the denture in place.

Removable partial dentures are among the most common prostheses for missing teeth, primarily because of their relatively lower cost when compared with fixed devices.

When you and your dentist are discussing types of artificial teeth, be sure to discuss each type's comparative advantages and disadvantages: cost, look, feel, in-chair preparation time and number of appointments to complete the work, durability, and risk of damage to surrounding healthy teeth. No matter which type of artificial teeth you choose, expect to make several visits to the dentist. Your remaining natural teeth must be cleaned of plaque and calculus; any decay and periodontal disease need to be treated before work on the prosthesis can begin. You may need other preparatory work as well. For example, neighboring teeth may have already begun to move into the space and need to be re-shaped or even moved orthodontically. Impressions of both jaws must be made so a study cast can be created to plan your treatment. Once supporting teeth have been prepared with crowns, notches and/or etched surfaces, final impressions are taken from which the artificial teeth will be made at a dental laboratory. For removable dentures, you'll try the framework for fit and have adjustments made to it before the artificial teeth are added, first temporarily for a fitting, and then permanently. You'll also have to return for adjustments during the first few months after your new partial denture is in place.

WHEN ALL YOUR NATURAL TEETH ARE LOST. Despite continuing efforts to develop "natural" dentures, including implants (see chapter 7), nothing surpasses natural teeth for fit and function.

Nevertheless, some developments in denture technology have been made to overcome a few of the problems associated with dentures, such as poor fit, cracks in the base material, gum sores and dislodging when laughing. The traditional denture, comprised of natural-colored plastic teeth in a pink plastic base, rests directly on your gum tissue and bone. It is held in place—sometimes not very well—by a thin film of saliva.

If you have several teeth with sound roots, however, you may be able to wear an overdenture. Looking the same as standard dentures, overdentures are held more securely in place by attaching to the specially prepared surface of these healthy roots. The tooth crowns are ground to the gum line, a root canal is performed to remove the nerve, and the remaining tooth surface is prepared either by being overlaid with gold or having a steel post inserted. The denture is then clipped onto the roots or has tiny magnets on its undersurface that are attracted to the steel. These overdentures give a more natural sensation when biting and chewing and are more stable than standard dentures. They also help decrease bone resorption so there is less change in your gum line over time. (Resorption is the loss of tissue, such as bone, by the breakdown of the tissue.) The only significant disadvantage is that the overdenture base is hard to clean and the retained roots are susceptible to decay.

You may also have the choice of delayed or immediate dentures. In the past, dentures were put into place six or more weeks after teeth were extracted, in the belief that gums needed to heal before bearing weight. While many people continue to wait, an increasing number are choosing to have their dentures put into place on the same day as the extraction. In addition to the obvious cosmetic benefit of avoiding a period of toothlessness, many people also find that their gums actually heal faster and with less pain when covered by the denture base than when left uncovered.

Immediate dentures actually involve several steps. Your back teeth are removed first and allowed to heal. Your dentist takes an impression and makes a cast from which your front teeth are removed. Once the lab completes your denture from the cast, your actual front teeth can be extracted and the denture put into place.

No matter what type of denture you choose, you will need ongoing dental care. Dentures are not a way to avoid going to the dentist. You'll need frequent adjustments to your dentures as your gum and bone recede, especially if you get immediate dentures. You'll still need care for your gums and may eventually need surgery to remove excess gum tissue that interferes with your dentures.

Agreeing to dentures is a significant health decision and is irreversible. Don't be pressured into a hasty decision by a dentist who insists, "You'll be better off without your teeth" or "These teeth aren't worth the cost of saving them." Carry out your own evaluation of need before you decide.

EVALUATING YOUR NEED FOR DENTURES. If periodontal disease has left your natural teeth so loose that you have difficulty chewing or if your teeth have been extensively damaged in an accident, then you may have little choice about whether to get dentures. If, however, you have some healthy teeth, still held firmly in your gums, then your options are greater.

Denturism: Yet Another Choice

Commonly, people needing dentures have their teeth extracted by an oral surgeon or general dentist, and then the dentist or a prosthodontist takes an impression and sends it off to a dental laboratory where the dentures are made. The dentist or prosthodontist fits them…and sends his rather substantial bill.

People living in Arizona, Colorado, Idaho, Maine, Montana, Oregon and Washington, however, have an alternative, one that could save them a lot of money and give them quality dentures. That alternative is denturism.

Denturists are technicians trained to fit and make dentures. In the seven states listed above, they are licensed by the state to work directly with patients. A dentist or oral surgeon still extracts the remaining natural teeth, but patients have the choice to work directly with the denturist, who takes the impression, makes the dentures and fits them.

To practice in these states, denturists must have the equivalent of two years of college and actual experience making dentures (the amount varies; in Colorado, for example, they must have at least 1,000 hours). The education may include courses in a dental hygiene or other allied dental program. Other denturists may have been educated in Canada, where the profession has a long history and several training programs are offered. Also, in 1997, plans were under way to open the Regional Denturist Education Program at Bates Technical College in Tacoma, Washington. Candidates for licensure must also successfully pass an examination that includes a written test and an actual procedure. As with other dental professionals, denturists' practice is overseen by a state board, either the same board that oversees dentists or a separate state board of denture technology.

Financial issues are a driving force for both supporters and opponents of denturism. In Oregon, which has had licensed

continued

denturism since the late 1970s, a 1991 study comparing costs of dentures purchased from dentists and denturists found that the average fee charged by the denturists was less than half that of the dentists. Not surprisingly, dentists strongly oppose licensing denturists. Senior citizen and other consumer groups are equally strong in their support.

For more information about denturism—and to find out if your state is among the 18 states that have denturist associations—contact the National Denturist Association at the following address:

> Wanda Anderson
> Executive Director
> National Denturist Association
> P.O. Box 637
> Poulsbo, WA 98370

Before agreeing to have all your teeth removed and dentures made, be sure you get at least one other professional opinion. In addition, ask about conservative measures that could delay your need for full dentures—again, can the teeth in the worst condition be extracted and a partial denture made? Finally, ask a lot of questions, among them:

1. **Who will extract my teeth? My general dentist? An oral surgeon?**

The number of teeth to be extracted, your general health, the need for general anesthesia and the perceived difficulty in removing your teeth are among the factors influencing the choice of dentist or oral surgeon (see also chapter 4). If two professionals are involved, be sure you know who will be responsible for any follow-up care for your gums. The last thing you want to hear when your gum is swollen and painful is your general dentist saying, "This isn't my responsibility. You'll have to see the oral surgeon."

2. How long are these dentures likely to last? Is there a written warranty?

The American Dental Association and other experts suggest that five years is a reasonable life span of a set of removable dentures. Your bone under the dentures will resorb and change the contour of your gum line so much by then that adjustments will no longer be effective.

3. How many appointments will be needed to prepare for the dentures and to properly fit them? Are these visits included in the fee?

You may need gum or bone surgery to remove irregularities before dentures can be made. In addition, once you're wearing dentures, several appointments will probably be needed for adjustments. Be sure to find out if there's a schedule (every three months, for example), how many visits are usual, what happens if your case is unusual and how these visits are handled in the fee.

Speaking of fees, be sure to get a written description of exactly what is included. If an oral surgeon will extract your teeth and your general dentist will make and fit your dentures, you need to get an itemized statement from both professionals. Take your time and read the itemization carefully. Are only a limited number of follow-up visits included? If so, how much will other visits cost? How much is for the denture itself and how much for the dentist's labor?

Dental Care in Nursing Homes

Entering a nursing home should not cut you off from dental care and good oral hygiene, but it does for most residents. Since 1987, federal regulations have required any nursing facility that receives Medicare or Medicaid funding to actively provide or obtain dental care for their residents. However, neither Medicare nor Medicaid covers most dental care (see chapter 8), so typically, payment for such services comes out of your pocket.

Federal law also requires nursing staff to carry out a comprehensive assessment within a few days of admission of the

continued

client's medical, psychological and dental needs. "Unfortunately, nursing staff often lack the training, equipment and time needed to carry out the oral health portion of the assessment effectively," conclude Michael J. Helgeson, D.D.S., and Barbara J. Smith, R.D.H., M.P.H., of the department of preventive sciences at the University of Minnesota School of Dentistry. Enforcement is weak, they add.

These deficiencies are also factors in the poor daily oral care that most nursing home residents receive. Many residents can't carry out their own oral hygiene unassisted and must rely on nurses, nurses aides or family members. As Helgeson and Smith write in their 1996 article in *Special Care in Dentistry,* "Poor daily oral care continues to be widespread and unchecked among most nursing home residents."

If you or a loved one faces a nursing home stay longer than three months, one of your concerns must be for oral care (short stays will have little, if any, permanent impact on your oral health). In 1996, a Consensus Conference on Developing Practice Guidelines for Institutionalized Older Dental Patients identified a number of indicators of quality dental care. While these are not binding on nursing homes or dentists and you certainly won't find a facility that achieves all of them, they can help you evaluate the current level of oral care a facility provides.

Signs of Quality Daily Oral Care

- The facility develops an oral care plan within 15 days of the patient's admission.
- The residents receive assistance as needed to carry out oral hygiene.
- The staff receive regular in-service training on daily oral care techniques.
- The staff consult with dentists, hygienists and physical therapists as needed to ensure that residents are able to carry out as much self-care as possible.

continued

■ The facility seeks feedback from visiting dentists during dental examinations about the effectiveness of daily care.

Some Signs of Quality Routine and Emergency Dental Care

■ The facility makes prompt referrals when dental emergencies arise.

■ The facility provides a staff member who coordinates on-site and off-site dental visits.

■ The facility provides an adequate work area if dental work is provided on site.

■ The staff assist with arranging medical consultations, communicating with family members and making financial arrangements, as needed, for dental care.

■ The staff receive regular in-service training on evaluating and responding to dental emergencies and providing follow-up care.

Nursing facilities usually contract with dentists and hygienists in the community to provide care as needed, although a few very large facilities may have one or more on staff. Ask for the list of providers and evaluate them as we suggested in chapter 1. Ask other residents about their satisfaction with the dental care and each dentist. Find out when the dentist and hygienist regularly visit the facility and meet them—before you need care. If care is provided on site in a mobile van or with mobile equipment the dentist brings and sets up in a room at the nursing facility, ask to see it as it is used with patients (or have a family member do this for you). Technological developments in equipment mean that dentists can bring a fully equipped operatory to the nursing home—you should not receive or accept lower quality care than that available in the dentist's office. Nor should restorative or oral surgical care be provided in anything less than a fully staffed and equipped operatory—mobile or office-based.

WHEN ILLNESS AFFECTS DENTAL CARE

At some stage in life, you or a loved one may be "medically compromised." That's what doctors and dentists call people whose health requires them to change their usual activities. Often, dental care is one of these activities.

Your status as a medically compromised patient may result from a physical or mental illness or a disability, whether the condition is temporary, has been present from birth or develops in adulthood and becomes chronic.

Among the temporary conditions are the following:

- Pregnancy
- Postoperative recuperation
- Cancer therapy
- Mild stroke, from which you completely recover
- Infectious diseases such as pneumonia or mononucleosis

Generally speaking, in such cases you may be able to postpone dental work until your condition improves. However, if the need is urgent—a tooth breaks, a filling falls out or your gums become inflamed, for example—you must get care.

Lifelong illnesses and disabilities present from birth offer enumerable challenges in everyday life. Among the conditions we might include are the following:

- Down syndrome and other forms of mental retardation
- Muscular dystrophy and other neuromuscular diseases
- Type 1 (insulin-dependent) diabetes mellitus
- Sickle-cell anemia
- Hemophilia and other bleeding disorders

In some instances, such as mental retardation, patients not only have difficulty understanding and agreeing to care, but they may also be unable to adequately carry out home care. Lack of care may combine with their medications' side effects and the effects of their illness on gums and teeth to cause significant periodontal disease, tooth decay and other dental problems that must receive care.

The third group of medically compromised patients develop a chronic illness, usually in adulthood, including:

- Heart disease
- Arthritis
- Type 2 (adult-onset) diabetes mellitus
- Emphysema and other lung diseases
- Cirrhosis, hepatitis and other liver diseases
- Acquired immune deficiency syndrome (AIDS)

These conditions may go for long periods without symptoms, only to flare up and cause acute illness. They put a heavy burden on the body's immune system and on other organs. As a result, people with chronic diseases often find themselves susceptible to major infections and illnesses that might be minor in healthy individuals, including complications from dental procedures, periodontal disease and stomatitis (mouth sores).

Before we explore some of the dos and don'ts of dental care for medically compromised patients, let's look in greater detail at how three illnesses and their therapy can affect your dental health.

Case: Coping With Cancer

Except for cancer of the mouth, which has a direct effect on teeth and gums, the harmful effects on your mouth related to cancer result primarily from the chemotherapy and radiation used to treat it. About 40 to 50 percent of patients receiving chemotherapy develop changes in their mouth, some of which are permanent. The mucosa that line your cheeks and gums can become inflamed and develop stomatitis. Your salivary glands don't produce enough saliva, a condition called xerostomia, which leads to tooth decay. Bacteria and viruses that normally live in your mouth without causing harm cause infections as your immune system becomes depressed from the toxic effects of the chemotherapy. People receiving radiation therapy, especially in the head and neck area, often develop permanent xerostomia, rapid tooth decay, stomatitis, slow wound healing and jaw pain. They are also susceptible to a condition called osteoradionecrosis in which the alveolar bone—the bony ridge of the jaw in which the tooth sockets are—disintegrates, especially after teeth are extracted.

If you have recently been diagnosed with cancer, in addition to the general dental guidelines given later in this chapter, here are some tips to lessen the impact of your therapy on your teeth and gums.

- If possible, before you undergo radiation therapy or chemotherapy, get a complete dental evaluation. Have your teeth professionally cleaned and any necessary dental work done.

- If you must have dental work done while undergoing chemotherapy, it should be scheduled when your red blood cell count is at its highest. Your dentist and oncologist (cancer specialist) should work together to plan the best times, usually just before another cycle of chemotherapy is due to begin.

- Large cancer centers have oncologists who provide dental care. If you wish to continue being cared for by your regular dentist, however, make sure he consults with your oncologist and/or the center's dental oncologist before providing your care.

- Help maintain your dental health during your illness through self-care: daily fluoride gel, gentle but thorough brushing and flossing (using foam-tipped pads when your red cell count is low) and frequent anti-bacterial mouth rinses—the most commonly prescribed techniques.

- Even after your chemotherapy and radiation therapy are over, the effects will linger and potentially affect your dental care. Make sure every dentist knows that you have had therapy, what kind and when it was given, and what part of your body underwent radiation. If you have had chemotherapy and you need oral surgery, your surgeon should consult with your oncologist before the procedure to make sure your red blood cell count has returned to normal.

Case: Type 1 Diabetes Mellitus

Type 1 diabetes mellitus, which used to be called juvenile-onset or insulin-dependent diabetes, is a complex disease with profound consequences on all aspects of your health. Diabetes also affects your oral health, especially when the disease is poorly controlled. Xerostomia is a common consequence of diabetes, as is glucose accumulation in the crevices around your teeth. Either condition contributes to higher-than-normal rates of tooth decay and periodontal disease. Wound healing is slow and your susceptibility to infection is increased. In turn, periodontal infections can contribute to insulin resistance, requiring you to take more insulin to control your disease.

Getting and maintaining control of your diabetes is, of course, the single most important factor in your dental health. That, however, is not always possible. Therefore, even diabetic people whose condition is currently under control need to plan their dental care as carefully as they monitor their blood glucose levels, with measures such as these:

- Have your physician provide your dentist with detailed information about your condition—when it was diagnosed, what medications you are taking and how, history of any complications and your latest blood glucose levels. Urge your physician and dentist to consult regularly before you receive dental care.

- If your diabetes is currently poorly controlled, avoid active dental treatment except for emergency care. Your dentist should consult with your physician and probably give antibiotics before emergency dental surgery. If your glucose levels fluctuate dramatically, you may need to have the surgery in a hospital with your physician in attendance to monitor your blood glucose levels.

- If your diabetes is under control, you can undergo routine dental procedures such as fillings without special precautions. However, if you must skip a meal before undergoing a dental procedure such as oral surgery, discuss with your physician how to adjust your insulin dose and if dietary supplementation with special nutritional liquids is necessary after surgery.

- Stress can bring on hypoglycemia, or insulin shock, a serious condition with symptoms of mental confusion, nausea, clammy skin and, if untreated, unconsciousness. Make sure your dentist knows the signs of hypoglycemia and what to do, including giving you orange juice, a soft drink or candy, followed by an injection of dextrose if you don't respond within a few minutes. To prevent shock, discuss with your dentist various stress-reduction techniques such as dividing procedures into segments that can be done over a number of appointments. Several other relaxation techniques are described in chapter 3.

For further information on how diabetes may affect your oral health or be affected by dental care, contact:

National Oral Health Information Clearinghouse
301-402-7364

National Institute of Dental Research
Information Office
Building 31, Room 2C35
31 Center Drive MSC 2290
Bethesda, MD 20892-2290
301-496-4261

Case: Heart Disease

Heart disease can actually manifest in any of a number of different conditions. Unlike many other conditions, heart disease itself has little direct effect on your oral health. However, you and your dentist must proceed with caution when planning any dental care, especially if your condition is newly diagnosed or unstable or you have recently undergone heart surgery. The American Heart Association and other experts suggest the following precautions for people needing dental care:

- If you suffer from almost any form of heart disease, but especially valve disease, you are more susceptible to endocarditis (infection of the heart lining). Therefore, most patients receive an antibiotic immediately before and just after dental procedures that cause bleeding. Bleeding allows the bacteria naturally in your mouth to enter the bloodstream and move toward your heart. Make sure your dentist knows before you visit about the details of your heart condition and consults with your physician about possible antibiotic therapy.

- The stress of a dental visit can put a strain on your heart, so you and your dentist should practice the stress-reduction techniques described in chapter 3 before and during your visit. This is particularly an issue for patients with angina. If you have stable angina, carry your nitroglycerine tablets with you to your dental visit and make sure your dentist knows what commonly triggers your attacks and what to do if one occurs: (1) Place you in an upright position; (2) put your nitroglycerine under your tongue; (3) give you oxygen; (4) monitor your blood pressure; (5) give you another tablet if you still have pain within five minutes; and (6) call in emergency assistance if pain persists for 10 minutes.

■ Only emergency dental care, with consultation between your dentist and physician, should be provided if your angina or other heart condition is unstable or you are recuperating from a heart attack or heart surgery. Dental care should be provided in the hospital, where constant monitoring and immediate emergency care are available.

■ If you are taking anticoagulant medication to prevent blood clots from forming in your heart or arteries, tell your dentist before you visit. She should consult with your physician about your current level of clotting and *measures to take during dental procedures to control bleeding.* For example, the dentist can apply a gelatin sponge to the area of bleeding and stimulate clotting only in that area. If a tooth has been extracted and, therefore, leaves a large bleeding area, the dentist can apply a soft plastic splint that applies gentle pressure to the wound to slow bleeding.

■ If you have a cardiac pacemaker, tell your dentist before she begins any procedure. Some electrical equipment, such as the TENS (transcutaneous electric nerve stimulation) device to provide electronic anesthesia, can damage or interfere with your pacemaker.

No matter what condition puts you into a medically compromised state, as a savvy dental consumer, your goal is to keep your oral health and your dental care from interfering with your recuperation, in the case of temporary illnesses, or with your successful adaptation to long-term conditions. In addition to the specific suggestions just described for three major illnesses, there are some general guidelines from which any medically compromised patient can benefit.

The Dos and Don'ts of Dental Care for Medically Compromised Patients

To get the best care, DO:

■ Look for a dentist with training, experience and interest in treating special patients. Dentists working at university clinics, dental specialists and general dentists who have completed a fifth year of dental education—postgraduate general dentistry—are most likely to have had training in caring for special needs patients (see chapter 1). Dentists with experience and interest are likely to know what questions to ask and to have office routines that decrease your risk of infection and make it easier for you to get care. They are aware that your medical history and diagnostic evaluation may take longer than for "nonspecial" people.

■ Keep your dentist informed about your medical condition. Your initial medical history may become quickly outdated and useless unless you update your dentist at each visit. Even a change in medication can significantly affect what your dentist can or can't do. Carry a list of current medications and verify the accuracy of your medication history in your dental record at each visit.

■ Make sure your dentist is comfortable consulting with your physician and vice versa. Change dentists (or physicians) if not. This is no time for professional jealousy, turf wars or other personal or professional characteristics that could interfere with your care. Provide each professional with the other's name, address and telephone number. Let them know that you expect them to consult as often as necessary on your care. If you need dental surgery or dental care in a hospital, discuss the advisability of having your physician assist (the hospital may require it).

■ Whenever your physician prescribes a drug, ask about side effects, including those that affect your teeth and gums. A 1994 study found that 80 percent of the 131 most frequently prescribed medications caused xerostomia and 34 percent brought on stomatitis. Urge your doctor to discuss drug side effects or other potential dental complications of your therapy with your dentist.

■ When you call for a dental appointment, remind the scheduling assistant about your condition. At the very least, she may need to allow extra time for the appointment to update your medical history or for procedure preparation. Furthermore, the dentist may need to consult with your physician and/or prescribe antibiotics before your visit.

■ If you are responsible for a disabled or medically compromised adult, encourage him or her to take as active a role in oral hygiene and dental care as possible. Insist that the dentist discuss treatment options with the patient. Ask about special devices such as toothbrushes with large handles for better gripping to help the patient carry out home care.

To get the best care, DON'T:

■ Ignore your dental health on the assumption that your teeth are much less important than your medical condition or disability. Faced with a serious disease or disability, you may understandably tend to overlook dental care. Infected gums, however, can introduce dangerous bacteria into your bloodstream and further deteriorate your health. Painful gums or teeth can prevent you from eating healthful foods, lowering both your quality of life and nutritional status. If teeth and gums are left to deteriorate, you may face oral surgery at a time when your body is already under stress.

■ Assume that your dentist knows the impact of dental procedures or drugs on your condition. As we've noted before, always ask about side effects before taking prescribed medications—ask your dentist, doctor or pharmacist. Remind the dentist about any past visits, for example, when you had difficulty breathing after she put you into a reclining position.

Buyer, Beware:
Issues of Dental Care

 n this chapter, we explore several areas of dentistry that have been the subjects of great controversy: the diagnosis and treatment of temporomandibular disorders; cosmetic dentistry; and implant surgery. We emphasize that each of these is a legitimate dental therapy with benefits to some patients. Read on to find out if you can truly benefit from developments in these areas.

TEMPOROMANDIBULAR DISORDERS

Perhaps no area of contemporary dentistry is as controversial as temporomandibular disorders (TMD). Experts seem to disagree over even the name for this group of disorders, as well as how they should be diagnosed and treated.

Only recently have careful studies been done to identify the symptoms that consistently differentiate TMD from other causes of pain and to demonstrate reliably the effectiveness of newer diagnostic tests and nonsurgical therapies. In preparing this section, we have reviewed reports of these recent studies; we present what is currently known, which differs significantly from what was thought just a few years ago. Research continues. Anyone diagnosed with TMD or experiencing the

symptoms we describe below needs to stay abreast of these ongoing research findings and to consult a dentist who does the same.

Do These Symptoms Have a Name?

One of the most basic disagreements among dental experts regarding the diseases that affect the temporomandibular (TM)
joint is just what to call them. Originally, the condition was
called Costen's syndrome after the physician who first described it. In the 1980s, temporomandibular joint syndrome
was the common term, with patients and the popular press often shortening this simply to TMJ. More recently, dental experts,
including the American Dental Association, refer to temporomandibular disorders (TMD), recognizing that several conditions produce similar symptoms. A few researchers argue that
the term myofascial pain dysfunction more accurately describes
the particular collection of symptoms, but this phrase has had
limited acceptance to date.

In this book, we use TMD in line with the present consensus. However, if you carry out your own research on the conditions, watch for these other terms as well.

What Are Temporomandibular Disorders?

One thing dental experts seem to agree on is that what was once considered a single disease is actually a collection of medical and dental
conditions. These conditions affect the temporomandibular (TM) joint—
the point at which the lower jaw (mandible) is joined to the skull (temporal bone)—and/or the muscles used in chewing and moving the jaw.

In the 1980s, TMD (or TMJ syndrome, as it was more commonly
called then) was a popular diagnosis for patients with a wide range of
symptoms that often defied any other diagnosis. These symptoms included headaches, earaches, dizziness, facial pain, locked jaw, abnormal

tooth wear, and clicking or popping sounds in the jaw. As a result of this use of TMD as a catchall diagnosis, estimates of the number of sufferers were 60 million or more in the United States alone.

Researchers have been making an effort to more precisely define TMD and to more accurately assess the number of sufferers. At present, the three primary signs and symptoms commonly associated with TMD are:

■ *Pain in the TM joint area, either when pressure is applied or when the jaw moves.* Facial pain, earache and neck pain are also reported. In what is probably the first large-scale population-based study of TMD in the United States, Samuel F. Dworkin, D.D.S., Ph.D., and colleagues at the University of Washington found that individuals diagnosed with TMD were four to six times more likely to have pain than normal study subjects when pressure was applied to the skin over the muscles of the lower jaw. Dworkin's report, published in 1990 in the *Journal of the American Dental Association,* also noted that about half of the TMD patients experienced pain when they chewed or bit down on a cotton roll.

■ *Abnormal jaw function (jaw dysfunction).* What constitutes normal jaw functioning has not been fully defined, but TM disorders often interfere with a person's ability to open her mouth fully without pain. Measuring from the tip of the upper central incisor to the lower one, the University of Washington group used 30 millimeters (1.2 inches) for females and 35 millimeters (1.4 inches) for males to define restricted opening. Twenty-two percent of patients being treated for TMD were unable to open their mouths wider than this defined level. In addition to restricted opening, some people with TMD may actually have their jaws lock either open or closed.

■ *Joint sounds on movement.* Unlike pain or restricted motion, clicking, popping or grating noises when the jaw moves do not interfere with jaw function or affect quality of life significantly. Nevertheless, these sounds have long been associated with a diagnosis of TMD. The University of Washington study found that joint clicks were present in 43 percent of patients with TMD; almost an equal percentage, however, had no distinguishable joint sounds at all. Less than 10 percent had a grating sound.

In a 1996 report, also published in the *Journal of the American Dental Association,* of a conference convened by the National Institute of Dental Research and the National Institutes of Health (NIH), the total number of TMD sufferers was estimated to be about 10 million. While men and women appear to suffer from TMD in about equal numbers, people

Finding Someone to Diagnose and Treat TMD

The diagnosis and treatment of TMD are not the exclusive purview of any one type of dentist or health care provider. Most commonly, general dentists, prosthodontists, orthodontists and oral surgeons are the professionals involved. Furthermore, because stress and other behavioral issues are closely associated with TMD, psychologists and psychiatrists often come into the picture. Referrals to physical therapists, neurologists, nutritionists, orthopedic surgeons, and ear, nose and throat specialists (otolaryngologists) are also not uncommon. Finally, some practitioners call themselves TMD specialists or myofascial surgeons, although there is no such professionally recognized or certified specialty.

Experience and qualifications are more important than any particular specialty or title when seeking someone to guide your diagnosis and treatment. If you suspect you have TMD and want to use a dental caregiver, try the following sources:

- Your general dentist, who may provide the care or give referrals to others who do
- Local pain clinics, which are becoming increasingly common in metropolitan areas and which offer a variety of pain-related services in one location
- Local dental society, which may provide referrals to individuals with experience treating TMD
- University dental schools, which may offer TMD clinics or referrals to dentists with TMD experience

seeking therapy are overwhelmingly women. The disorders are most common in people ages 20 to 40, although children and older adults are also found to have TMD.

If you suspect that you or someone you know may have TMD, the first step is to try to get an accurate diagnosis.

How Are Temporomandibular Disorders Diagnosed?

Although numerous efforts have been made to find electronic or other tools to objectively diagnose TMD (as we describe on page 202), very few have been proven accurate and valid. Therefore, according to Norman Mohl, D.D.S., Ph.D., of the State University of New York at Buffalo, and others, the best available means for diagnosis remains a careful and thorough history and examination, supported in some cases by TM joint imaging. Specifically, your dentist should carry out the following:

■ A complete history that includes questions about your symptoms, factors that affect those symptoms (for example, less pain when you apply hot compresses), timing of symptoms (both when they began and times when they are more or less intense) and restrictions your symptoms have imposed. You also need to bring your dentist up to date on your medical history with information on current medications you're taking, illnesses and conditions you're being treated for and the results of any medical tests you've recently had. (A number of chronic illnesses such as arthritis are associated with TMD.) You also need to discuss your recent family, psychosocial and behavioral history because stress is a common factor in the development of TMD.

■ A physical examination that includes an inspection of your head and neck and an assessment of the range of motion of your lower jaw— side-to-side movement, up and down, with and without pain. The dentist uses a millimeter ruler to measure how wide you can open your mouth. The physical also includes what is called muscle and joint palpation. Simply put, this means he feels your facial muscles and TM joint both while you are still and you move your jaw. He may use a pressure algometer device that allows him to apply consistent pressure to about a dozen sites along your jaw, around your ear and on your forehead. This handheld device has a calibrated pressure gauge attached to a short rod.

The dentist manually applies one to two pounds of pressure and notes when pain occurs.

Another part of the physical examination is an assessment of joint sounds, which is the subject of considerable controversy for two reasons. First, research has found that an examiner's ability to accurately detect and distinguish the various types of sounds is unreliable. A study by researchers at the University of Washington, for example, found that even when examiners were given supervised training on evaluation techniques, including joint sound detection using both a stethoscope and feeling with their fingertips (palpation) as joints moved, their reliability in detecting and identifying types of sounds ranged from marginally acceptable to poor. A second area of controversy is just what diagnostic value, if any, joint sounds have. As we've noted, about 43 percent of people diagnosed with TMD have clicking sounds when they move their jaws. However, almost an equal number have no sound at all. Furthermore, as Mohl points out in a 1994 *Journal of the American Dental Association* article, "TMJ clicking is exceedingly common in the [general] population, may be caused by a variety of mechanisms, is usually not permanent and does not necessarily imply that serious sequelae [disease] will follow."

The physical examination also includes an examination inside your mouth. In particular, the dentist is looking for evidence of bruxism— i.e., grinding or clenching your teeth repeatedly. Often unconscious, this habit results in irregular wear of enamel on biting surfaces and can even loosen teeth. Although bruxism is commonly associated with TMD, it is unclear whether bruxism is a cause or an effect.

- Tests using various imaging techniques in selected patients. Guidelines have not been developed to clearly identify patients who should or should not undergo x-rays or other imaging tests to diagnose TMD. Mohl and others suggest that patients whose symptoms developed after an injury to the head or neck, who have significant loss of jaw function or recent changes in occlusion, or whose symptoms and history suggest a problem with the TM joint itself are candidates for imaging tests. Patients who have joint sounds without pain or jaw dysfunction will not benefit from these tests.

Considerable controversy arises over just which imaging test or tests should be used. Among the current candidates are:

Panoramic x-ray, a radiation-based image, taken with a special machine, that shows all the teeth and surrounding bone on one large piece of x-ray film. Panoramic x-rays are probably of the greatest value to the greatest number of people, according to experts.

Computed tomography (CT), a radiation-based technique that uses multiple, simultaneous x-ray beams to produce a cross-sectional view highlighting the bones and soft tissues of the jaw and head. Computed tomography is most useful in showing bone fractures and degeneration of bone caused by arthritis or other degenerative joint diseases.

Arthrography, a radiation-based technique in which a dye is injected into the TM joint and both moving and still x-rays are taken

Magnetic resonance imaging (MRI), a technique that uses radio frequency waves to produce cross-sectional views of tissues surrounding the jawbone and TM joint

Arthrography, MRI and CT can show irregularities in the TM joint itself; however, at present, those irregularities don't appear to be related to pain or joint dysfunction in most patients, so identifying the problem doesn't aid diagnosis or treatment. Tumors in the TM joint region are "exceedingly rare," according to studies cited by James Howard, D.D.S., in a 1990 *California Dental Association Journal* article. If such a tumor is suspected, CT and MRI are the best imaging alternatives.

In addition to the issue of usefulness, each of these tests brings other concerns as well. The radiation-based tests must be evaluated in terms of safety and exposure to radiation (see chapter 2). Arthrography is a technically difficult test to perform, requiring a highly skilled technician. Interpreting CT scans and MRI views of the TM joint region is difficult and requires an experienced radiologist to accurately assess the results. All of these tests add to the cost of care, especially MRI, which is the most expensive of the alternatives.

Using Electronics to Diagnose TMD

Like their medical counterparts, dentists are not immune to the lure of gadgets. That, combined with the legitimate need for objective methods to diagnose TMD, is a compelling force in the appearance of various electronic devices in dental offices that treat TMD. Among the devices you are most likely to see are:

- **Surface electromyograph (EMG),** which uses patch electrodes placed over the chewing muscles to record the muscles' electrical output at rest and moving, much as an EKG measures the heart muscle
- **Sonograph,** which measures intensity, duration and frequency of sounds made by the moving jaw
- **Mandibular kinesiograph (jaw tracking),** which attempts to measure the movement patterns of the jaw using a magnet attached to the lower incisors and magnetic sensors on various locations of the face

These tests are noninvasive, involve little pain except that caused by jaw movement and can be performed in a dentist's office without anesthesia. However, some researchers have concluded that there is little or no evidence that any of these tests are of any real value in diagnosing TMD. Researchers from McGill University, the University of Florida and the University of Montreal, for example, evaluated these devices and concluded that "the use of these instruments in clinical practice is inappropriate at this time." According to their 1995 report in the *Journal of Dental Research,* many of the tests have high false-positive results—i.e., they often indicate that people have TMD when they don't.

Undergoing these tests will increase your dental costs, subject you to potential misdiagnosis and possibly delay treatment while you wait for tests and their results. Use the questions on the following page to evaluate *any* test your dentist suggests to diagnose temporomandibular disorders.

Given the uncertainty that exists among dental experts over the ultimate value of these tests, you need to be particularly wary of their use. Before you agree to any test, ask:

1. Why do you want to use this test rather than another in my case?

2. What do you expect the test to tell you that you don't already know?

3. If the results are inconclusive, what will the next step be?

4. How do you plan to use the results?

5. How will my treatment differ with the test results versus without them?

6. What is the rate of false negatives (the results indicate you are free of a disease when you in fact are not)?

7. What is the rate of false positives (the results indicate you have a disease when you don't)?

8. Can we proceed with treatment without this test?

How Are Temporomandibular Disorders Treated?

Treatment of TMD is yet another area of professional controversy. What dental experts can agree on is the need with most patients to try conservative, noninvasive, reversible therapies before resorting to surgery or major orthodontic therapy.

NONSURGICAL THERAPY. In its 1996 report, the NIH conference panel concluded that for many people, these disorders are self-limiting. In other words, over time the conditions (or at least the symptoms) disappear. Thus, the NIH panel and others suggest conservative therapies first to relieve the pain and joint dysfunction. The panel also points out that very few reliable, well-designed studies have been carried out testing the effectiveness of one therapy over another or even of just a "wait and see" approach. The NIH report notes, "Diagnosis and initial treatment often depend on the practitioner's experience and philosophy, rather than on scientific evidence."

If you are diagnosed with TMD, this means that you must be wary of anyone who promises instant results, guarantees relief or urges costly orthodontic therapy or reconstruction that involves replacing all your existing crowns and bridges with new ones, as your first or only alternative. As we've emphasized throughout this book, question why a particular therapy is recommended, what results to expect and what your alternatives are, including what may happen if you do nothing. Further, you may also need to try more than one therapy to get relief from your symptoms.

Among your nonsurgical choices for treatment are:

■ **Behavioral techniques,** including hypnosis to eliminate bruxism or other destructive oral habits, stress management training and biofeedback. Dental experts agree that stress and muscle tension are major factors in TMD development.

■ **Drug therapy,** which usually involves pain relief with nonsteroidal anti-inflammatory drugs, such as over-the-counter ibuprofen, and can include muscle relaxants or even low-dose antidepressant drugs. Drug therapy is usually used in combination with other techniques because it only relieves pain and does nothing to change any underlying cause.

■ **Physical therapy,** which involves regular exercises of the jaw, initially under the supervision of a physical therapist

■ **Transcutaneous electric nerve stimulation (TENS),** which uses a low-level electrical current to relax the jaw muscles and reduce pain. Dental experts disagree over the device's ability to actually move the mandible when a more intense current is applied and thus correct misalignment that may cause TMD.

■ **Splints, called occlusal, bite or stabilization splints,** involving the use of an acrylic removable mouthpiece in the upper and lower jaws. The splints are worn 24 hours a day for up to six months, during which time the jaw alignment is temporarily adjusted. Once the person has been without pain for up to three months, the splints are removed during the daytime, but continue to be used in the upper jaw at night indefinitely.

■ **Bite adjustment, also known as occlusal equilibration,** in which the dentist uses his high-speed handpiece and an abrasive tip to selectively remove very thin layers from the chewing surface of teeth. Removing irregularities that affect how the two jaws meet can quickly correct TMD in some people.

- **Orthodontics,** which is the most drastic of the nonsurgical options. Because the effects are irreversible, the cost is high and TMD symptoms may not be eliminated, orthodontic treatment to realign the bite is very rarely a first-choice TMD therapy. However, if other measures fail, this may be one of the few alternatives available.

SURGICAL THERAPY. Only a small percentage—1 to 5 percent—of patients with TMD are candidates for surgery. Among the reasons to consider surgery are moderate to severe pain not relieved by other therapies, jaw dysfunction that significantly affects the patient's quality of life, evidence of a tumor or what surgeons call "joint derangement," the latter a situation in which a disk at the tip of the joint is out of place. Degenerative joint disease such as rheumatoid arthritis, in which the bones of the joint degenerate and affect movement, may also call for surgery. Nevertheless, remember: Surgical therapy remains controversial. Research has not been done to establish the effectiveness of most therapies or to compare one procedure with another.

Surgical procedures for TMD range from arthroscopy to total joint replacement. Briefly, the following are the two main types.

- **Arthroscopy.** With the patient under general anesthesia, the surgeon makes a small incision just in front of the ear and uses slender instruments connected to a video camera and monitor to examine the joint area, remove debris or damaged tissue and possibly to adjust alignment of the disk or condyle.

- **Open arthroplasty.** Several procedures fall within this general category, and in each the surgeon opens the area around the joint for full view without video equipment. These procedures allow greater visibility and maneuverability for the surgeon than does arthroscopic surgery. Therefore, the open procedures are most likely to be used to remove or repair the disk, to remove bony growths from the back side of the condyle or fossa or to correct perforation of the jawbone into the temporal bone.

A Warning About Disk Replacement Surgery

When a torn or degenerated disk is the cause of TM joint pain or dysfunction, an oral surgeon may have to remove the disk in a procedure called a diskectomy. Although many patients are satisfied with the results without a replacement for the disk, evidence of degeneration of the joint over a period of years has led many dental experts to recommend a disk implant during the diskectomy.

In the mid-1980s, thousands of patients received alloplastic implants—that is, disk replacements made from inert plastic. In a 1995 article in *Medical Care,* Alexia Antczak-Bouckoms, D.M.D., Sc.D., M.P.H., of Tufts University School of Medicine, says these implants "were introduced, granted Food and Drug Administration approval and widely used without the benefit of human or animal testing."

Although initially successful, over time the implants began to break down, causing destruction of the TM joint itself and the need for a second surgical procedure to replace the implant.

If you have been diagnosed with disk damage severe enough to warrant diskectomy, you do have alternatives to an alloplastic implant. Discuss this issue with your dentist and oral surgeon. Get a second and even a third opinion before proceeding with this delicate surgery.

Both arthroscopy and arthroplasty are susceptible to the risks of other oral surgical procedures (see chapter 4) and of general anesthesia (see chapter 3). In particular, risks include infection, damage to nerves and other neighboring structures and failure to correct TMD. Before undergoing TM surgery, these questions should be among the ones you ask your surgeon.

1. **What experience have you had with this procedure?**
2. **What nonsurgical therapies are applicable in this situation?**

3. What are the likely consequences of delaying surgery for six months or a year?

4. Why are you recommending this procedure over another?

5. What are the risks associated with the procedure? In particular, what complications have your patients had and with what results?

6. Can I speak with another patient who has undergone the same procedure?

7. What has been the success rate in your patients with the recommended procedure?

8. What percentage of your patients return after a year or more with recurrence of TMD symptoms?

In order to get the most appropriate and effective care, ask plenty of questions and arm yourself with knowledge. Remember, too, that for many people temporomandibular disorders correct themselves over time.

COSMETIC DENTISTRY

Cosmetic dentistry refers to procedures done solely to improve appearance. This distinguishes these techniques from many dental procedures that *primarily* cure dental disease or restore function but may also take appearance into account. For example, an artificial crown restores function. But choosing a porcelain crown over a gold one to replace a broken incisor is a cosmetic (or aesthetic) decision because either crown would restore function.

Most dentists today have healthier patients who need fewer fillings and crowns than patients in the past. So cosmetic dentistry is a boon for dentists, especially general dentists. Editorials and commentaries in dental journals urge dentists to build their practice income by increasing the number of cosmetic procedures they perform. These procedures are paid for entirely by patients because insurance and managed care plans don't cover elective procedures. As one dental practice management consultant has written, "Elective [cosmetic] dentistry must become the wave of the future boutique practice."

True, there are legitimate reasons for undergoing the cosmetic dental procedures, but those reasons should be the patient's, not the dentist's. Aside from orthodontics (see chapter 5), which may be performed for purely cosmetic reasons, here are the three most common cosmetic procedures.

Bleaching

Teeth become discolored for a variety of reasons, some of which can be corrected with a bleaching process. If teeth are discolored by stains from tea, coffee or tobacco, excessive fluoride use, aging or antibiotics use, especially tetracycline or minocycline, bleaching may lighten the stains. If the tooth is discolored because of internal decay, a dead nerve or corroded amalgam filling, bleaching will not help. In addition, yellow, orange and brown stains tend to bleach out better than gray, blue or mottled ones.

Bleaching can be done at the dentist's office or at home. The in-office procedure uses a 35 percent hydrogen peroxide gel or solution. The teeth to be bleached are cleaned of plaque and surface stains, and the person's gums are coated with petroleum jelly. Peroxide is applied to the teeth either directly or by wrapping them in peroxide-saturated gauze. The solution is activated by exposing it to 120° to 125°F heat. Then all materials are carefully removed, the patient brushes her teeth with a soft brush and mild toothpaste, and the dentist gently polishes the teeth. Up to 70 percent of discoloration may be removed at the first visit, but usually several visits, spaced four to six weeks apart, are needed to achieve the desired results. Furthermore, depending on the cause, the procedure may need to be repeated in a few years.

Dentist-monitored at-home bleaching has been in use since the end of the 1980s. The dentist creates a plaster mold of the teeth to be bleached and has a soft plastic mouthpiece made at the laboratory. The patient applies a 10 percent carbamide peroxide solution to the tray of the mouthpiece and wears it for several hours a day for two or more weeks. According to a study of this at-home technique, 62 percent of people retained satisfactory color after three years. Longer studies have not been done, nor have studies been done that compare in-office and at-home techniques.

Over-the-counter bleaching kits are available for use without dentist monitoring. However, the bleaching solution has a lower concentration of peroxide than the dentist-monitored gel does. The solution is also thinner, so it tends to leak more from the mouthpiece, which has not been custom-fitted. These factors combine to make the results even less predictable than with other bleaching methods.

Of the millions of bleaching procedures performed, the only side effects noted to date have been temporary gum irritation and tooth sensitivity to cold food or drink. However, not all stains can be removed. And stains may be removed unevenly. With in-home bleaching, some patients have also experienced stomach upset from swallowed peroxide and jaw soreness from excessive use of the mouthpiece. None of these techniques has been in use long enough to establish long-term effects, especially of repeated use.

Bonding

Bonding refers to the use of composite resin, a tooth-colored plastic, to improve a tooth's appearance. In particular, bonding can repair chips or cracks in teeth, rebuild edges to fill in small spaces between teeth, re-contour a tooth to make it appear aligned or cover discoloration.

The dentist applies a mild acid solution to the tooth surface to be bonded. This removes a very thin layer of enamel and leaves a microscopically irregular surface. The dentist then applies the composite resin, which adheres to the roughened surface. After shaping the composite resin into natural contours, the dentist exposes it to 20 to 60 seconds of a curing light wand that helps set the composite resin. The tooth is then smoothed and polished.

Composite resin is subject to staining, chipping and cracking. If it is used near the gum line, it can cause chronic gum irritation and redness. While improvements continue to be made, at present the composite resin becomes worn and needs to be replaced every few years.

Porcelain Veneers

Veneers involve cementing thin custom-made, tooth-colored pieces of porcelain onto a tooth's surface. While composite resin can be used as a veneer over the entire front surface of a tooth, porcelain is by far the more common material at present. Porcelain retains its color and resists staining and scratching better than composite resin does. It also adheres to the underlying tooth with about twice the strength of composite resin.

Veneering can change the outward appearance of a tooth, making it whiter, more even and larger to fill small spaces between teeth. It can also create the illusion of a slight change in position. Thus, it can be a solution for front teeth that are discolored, pitted, cracked, slightly misaligned or irregularly spaced.

Veneers are applied much like artificial fingernails. The tooth surface is etched with a mild acid solution, after which a cast is made. A laboratory makes the porcelain veneer from the cast. At a second appointment, the dentist cements the veneer to the tooth.

A one-visit process has recently been introduced that uses computer technology to enable the dentist to fabricate the veneer within minutes. Using a small, handheld camera, the dentist scans the surface of the tooth to be veneered. These images are fed into a computer, which creates the design for the veneer. A block of porcelain is placed in the unit's milling chamber, and the computer guides the sculpturing of the veneer. Within a few minutes, a rough veneer is ready to be cemented, then contoured and polished.

Veneers have been in widespread use only about a dozen years, and careful clinical studies of them are virtually nonexistent. However, experience has shown that porcelain veneers can be expected to last about five years. While they rarely delaminate (fall off), they do fracture with pressure, especially at the edges, and are difficult to repair. The veneer also thickens the tooth slightly, which can cause irritation along the gum line.

Veneers are not for everyone, so discuss with your dentist whether you are an ideal or unsuitable candidate.

Shopping for Cosmetic Dentistry

To avoid disappointment with or complications from a cosmetic dental procedure, shop carefully for a dentist to carry it out. Avoid being pressured into trying the latest gadget or technique with mere assurances that "it's harmless." Throughout this book, we've encouraged you to question, to get second opinions and to be an informed partner in your dental care. This is equally true when facing decisions about cosmetic dentistry. Here are some questions to ask your dentist before you decide to undergo cosmetic dentistry.

1. How long have you been performing this procedure?

These techniques are recent developments, and newer ones are always being introduced. So even an experienced practitioner may only have a few years' experience.

2. What training in this procedure have you had?

Commonly, dentists learn these techniques at workshops sponsored by the company that manufactures the bleaching kits, computerized veneer units or other devices to carry out the particular procedure. Professionals who are serious about learning these procedures and safely applying them will seek out other opportunities at workshops given by medical schools, the American Academy of Esthetic Dentistry and other professional organizations.

3. What can I reasonably expect the outcome to be?

Unrealistic expectations for results set you up for disappointment. Only with a good idea of the expected results can you effectively weigh the costs and risks against the outcome in order to make an informed decision.

4. What are the complications associated with this procedure? How many of your patients have experienced them?

A safe, effective procedure performed by an inexperienced or careless professional can easily become unsafe or ineffective. For example, the bonding process requires very careful technique, especially with regard to the "curing" step, to ensure adherence of the composite resin.

5. What are my alternatives to achieve the results desired?

If your dentist offers only one alternative, satisfy yourself that it is for a sound dental reason and not because this happens to be the only cosmetic procedure he knows.

DENTAL IMPLANTS

Dental implants are devices placed under the gum to which artificial teeth are attached. Implants can be and are used to replace a single tooth, but much of the current interest revolves around using implants with full upper or lower dentures (see chapter 6).

Implants are not new; some people have had them nearly 30 years. In 1982, however, Swedish researchers introduced North American dentists to a titanium implant with special qualities. Researchers had discovered in the early 1960s that when titanium was surgically implanted in bone, it wasn't rejected. More important, it allowed the bone tissue to grow up against it, which scientists call osseointegration. Other implanted metals in use at the time were also rarely rejected, but instead of being integrated into the bone, they were surrounded by softer, fibrous tissue that caused the implant to loosen over time and have to be removed. Osseointegrated titanium was held tightly in the bone, almost literally becoming a part of the bone, an important feature for a denture-anchoring device.

Dentists—and many of their patients—eagerly accepted this new technology. A study from the Harvard School of Dental Medicine found a 73 percent increase in the number of implants placed between 1986 and 1990. "Implantology" had come of age.

If you look beyond the hype, you may indeed find that implants are a suitable dental therapy for you. On the other hand, careful analysis may identify another alternative that fits your need—only you can choose.

The Types of Dental Implants

Dental implants come in three main forms. The first type, an endosseous implant, is surgically inserted into the bone. Endosseous implants are the most commonly used implants for all types of cases.

The second type, a subperiosteal implant, is comprised of a custom-fitted titanium framework that is surgically inserted under the gum, resting over the jawbone. It is predominantly used with patients whose jawbone is too thin or irregularly shaped to allow insertion of an implant directly into the bone.

The third type combines elements of the other two. Cylinders are inserted in the bone, and a bar or plate lies on top of the bone to connect them. This type, called a transosteal implant, is primarily used as an anchor for overdentures on the lower jaw. Overdentures are removable, so they are easier to clean than fixed dentures. For this reason, transosteal implants are often selected by people who have disabilities that could interfere with cleaning fixed dentures. Also, overdentures are less expensive to make than fixed dentures, so some people choose them to help control the cost of implants.

Who Performs Implant Surgery?

First, there is no certified specialty of "implantology," although you may find listings in your telephone directory for dentists calling themselves implantologists. Using the term may indicate the dentist's interest in performing implants or even his intention of limiting his practice to implant surgery, but it does not automatically indicate that he is any more qualified than any other dentist.

Implant procedures actually have two parts, each of which is often performed by a different type of dentist. The implant surgery is performed by oral surgeons, periodontists and, less frequently, general dentists. The prosthesis that attaches to the implant is fitted and installed by general dentists, prosthodontists or orthodontists.

The two dentists must work closely together if the final prosthesis is to have a perfect fit. The dentist making the prosthesis will be the one to provide the cast from which the surgeon will locate the implants. Because different types and brands of implants have variations in design and construction, both professionals must know in advance the type you will have so that the components of the implant and prosthesis will fit together. The surgeon is the one to help you evaluate your suitability for implants.

Among the possible sources to get names of specialists to perform implant surgery and fit the prosthesis are your local dental society, university dental schools, other patients who have undergone the procedure and your general dentist.

When dentists speak of implants, of course, they are referring to these metal supports. From the patient's perspective, however, there is another component: the crown, bridge or denture that will be attached to the implant. Generally speaking, these don't look much different from traditional prostheses. In fact, the casting and fitting process is much the same, as are the materials used. If the prosthesis is a removable overdenture, however, it will have tiny metal fasteners on the underside that align with the implants to allow the patient to insert and remove the denture several times a day for cleaning. If the prosthesis is a fixed style, it will have one or more holes through which tiny screws attach to the implant. Once the prosthesis is placed and adjusted, these holes are filled with composite resin. Should it be necessary to remove the prosthesis for adjustment or replacement, the dentist removes the composite resin and uses the holes to access the fasteners.

Implants Aren't for Everyone

Before a decision can be made about having implant surgery, all patients undergo a medical and dental history, clinical and x-ray examinations and an evaluation of a diagnostic plaster cast made of their jaws. The dentist needs to determine the following:

1. **Will the patient's health interfere with the placement of the implant or its long-term retention?**

    People with uncontrolled diabetes, bleeding disorders such as hemophilia, immune system diseases such as AIDS, or other conditions known to interfere with wound healing or cause surgical complications are not good candidates for implants.

2. **Are the person's gums and jawbone healthy and shaped so as to allow implantation?**

    Any sign of infection must be treated before surgery. Furthermore, the implants must be inserted at precise angles and in specific locations on the jaw in order to bear the pressure of biting and chewing without breaking or loosening. This means that patients with angled jaws or very irregular gum lines are not good candidates for implants.

3. **Does the bite line up well between any natural teeth that will remain in the area opposite the implant and the implant itself?**

An irregular bite puts heavy stress on the implant and may cause it to weaken or break, especially since natural teeth generate greater force than dentures.

4. Does the person understand the need for hygiene and follow-up, and is she capable of carrying out such a regimen?

In addition to regular dental visits to make adjustments and watch for infections or other problems, implants require meticulous oral hygiene to prevent infection, bone damage and loss of the implant.

As long as a patient is in good health, age is not a factor in the decision to have dental implants. Young or old, however, patients need to be highly motivated to have implants because of the numerous procedures, time and cost involved. As we describe in the next section, it can take six or more months to complete the process from evaluation to installation of the prosthesis.

The primary reason patients undergo implant surgery is for the stability the system gives to prostheses. Many patients, especially with fixed dentures, describe them as almost like natural teeth. The upper denture doesn't need a plate over the palate as traditional dentures do, so the speech difficulties that some patients experience are eliminated. Other patients who have difficulty adapting to dentures, for example, who gag or can't seem to keep the prosthesis in place during eating or speaking, seldom have difficulty adapting to dental implants.

At the end of this chapter, we give you a list of questions to ask to determine if implants are right for you. First, however, let's look at implant surgery.

Implant Surgery: What to Expect

Implant surgery must be performed in a sterile environment to prevent bacteria and other infectious agents from getting into the exposed bone. The setting may be a hospital or outpatient surgery center (see chapter 2). Less frequently, it can be a dentist's office, but it must be comparably equipped to the surgery center/hospital.

Surgical procedures vary somewhat depending on the type of implant being inserted. The most common implant currently in use is the endosseous cylinder.

With the patient under local anesthesia, the surgeon determines placement of the implants, often using a transparent plastic version of the diagnostic prosthesis made from the cast taken during the preliminary evaluation. At the site of the implant, she makes an incision into the gum tissue and slowly drills a hole into the bone. The cylinder implant core is screwed into the hole until the top is about even with the bone surface. A protective cap is added, then the gum tissue is sutured (stitched) back over the bone and implant core.

In about two weeks, the incision is healed enough to permit removal of the sutures. At this time, if the patient has a previous denture or had a temporary one made, it can be used for appearance. However, only soft food should be eaten, and most dentists advise patients to remove the denture whenever possible. In order for osseointegration (see page 212) to take place successfully, no pressure should be put on the implant during this early stage. Osseointegration of the implant into the bone takes about three to six months in the lower jaw, four to eight months in the upper jaw where the bone is softer and less dense.

The dentist periodically examines the implant and x-rays the jaw to determine if and when osseointegration has taken place. At that point, a second surgery is performed to reopen the gum tissue and expose the top of the implant core. The surgeon removes the temporary cover and inserts a titanium cylinder with a tiny protruding head into the core. Healing caps are put onto the cylinder head as a temporary measure while the gum heals around the cylinder, which takes an additional two to three weeks.

Insertion of the subperiosteal implant also involves two stages. During the first, the surgeon makes an incision in the gum tissue, exposing the jawbone. An impression of the bone ridge is made, and the incision is sutured. A laboratory makes the metal framework, which is comprised of a series of curved struts that lie over the bone and from which several posts protrude. When the framework is ready, the surgeon once again opens the gum and lays the implant over the bone. When the gum is sutured closed, the posts remain visible. Once the gum has healed and the underlying connective tissues have grown around the struts, the patient is ready for the final denture, which will attach to the protruding posts.

No matter what type of implant is used, healing should be complete before the final prosthesis is made and inserted. The dentist takes an impression in which the locations of the implants are marked and a cast is made. A crown or bridge is made, and in the case of dentures, the prosthesis that is made from the cast includes a metal framework for fastening to the implant, acrylic resin teeth and gum-colored acrylic resin on the front side to hide the area of attachment. At least two visits are needed for the prosthesis stage, to make the impression and to fit the final piece. Adjustment visits may also be needed; in addition, most patients with fixed prostheses, rather than removable ones, need to visit their dentist about every three months for regular cleaning and attachment checkups.

Evaluating Implants

If you are considering implants as part of a tooth replacement procedure, carefully interview your dentist and oral surgeon. Get a second and even a third opinion. Before making your final decision about proceeding, you need answers.

1. **In my particular case, why would you suggest implants?**

2. **Which type of implant do you recommend for me and why?**

3. **Approximately how many implants of each type have you done?**

Because of the popularity of cylindrical endosseous implants, the chances are that most surgeons' experience will be greater with them than with the other types. However, someone who has done only one or two of an implant type lacks sufficient experience for you to evaluate his expertise. When researchers at the University of Toronto analyzed the long-term results with cylindrical implants in patients with no teeth (edentulous), one conclusion in their 1996 report in the *Journal of the American Dental Association* was that most of the problems their patients experienced with broken implants or prosthetic frameworks were the result of inexperience on the part of the surgeon.

4. **What training have you had in implant placement and preparing prostheses for implants?**

Dentists training to become oral and maxillofacial surgeons, periodontists and prosthodontists do course work and usually gain some experience in placing and restoring implants. A few new programs are available for specialists to get an additional specialization in implant surgery. However, most dentists who carry out implant procedures learn their skills from the manufacturers of implant systems and from continuing education courses given by universities and private organizations such as dental laboratories.

5. What has been your success rate with this procedure?

Researchers at the Mayo Clinic using the cylindrical implant have reported a 98 percent success rate for implants in the lower jaw and 89 percent in the upper jaw after more than six years. Others have noted a five-year success rate of between 87.5 and 96.5 percent for the lower jaw and 81 percent for the upper jaw. An overall success rate with the transmandibular implant has been reported between 95.8 and 97.8 percent. Dale E. Smith, D.D.S., M.S.D., of the University of Washington School of Dentistry, and George A. Zarb, B.Ch.D., D.D.S., M.S., of the University of Toronto Faculty of Dentistry, have concluded that success rates of 85 percent at the end of five years and 80 percent at the end of 10 years are minimum levels of success for endosseous implants.

6. What complications might I encounter with implants?

Possible complications include infection of the gum tissue surrounding the implants, loosening of the implant that causes pain and problems with the prosthesis, breakage of one or more components of the implant or prosthesis, nerve damage resulting in facial numbness, speech difficulties associated with upper denture implants and a poorly aligned prosthesis as a result of poor implant placement.

7. Can I speak with another patient who has undergone the same procedure?

8. What alternatives are available to me if I choose not to have an implant?

Implant surgery is not emergency surgery. You can take your time, get all the facts you can, talk to patients and dentists. You can even decide to undergo traditional prosthetic therapy and keep implant surgery as an alternative in case you are dissatisfied with that therapy.

8

The Finances of Dental Care

elping you get the information you need to make wise dental choices is what this book is all about, and that includes how you'll finance the dental care you need. While cost should not be the deciding factor in the care you get, for most people, the issue of money cannot be ignored completely. In particular, if you have dental insurance, knowing your benefits before you need them can help you get the most for your dental dollar. On the other hand, if you are uninsured, identifying possible funding sources may influence where and when you get care, as we'll discuss later in this chapter. But first, let's look at the current state of affairs for those with dental insurance.

WHEN DENTAL CARE IS COVERED BY INSURANCE

About 46 percent of the U.S. population had dental benefits as of 1996, most often as part of their employers' benefits packages. An estimated 88 percent of employers provide some dental coverage, although employers with fewer than 500 employees are significantly less likely to do so than those with 2,500 to 4,999 workers, according to surveys. Those benefits are usually provided under one of two types of plans—traditional indemnity (also called fee-for-service) or managed care.

The Language of Dental Insurance

Your evaluation of your dental insurance options will be easier if the meanings of key terms are fresh in your mind.

- **Coinsurance.** This is the portion of the dental fees that must be paid by the consumer. In many plans, for example, the insurance company pays 80 percent of the fee for fillings and the consumer pays 20 percent. (Coinsurance is sometimes used interchangeably with the term *copayment*. But to be completely accurate, copayment should refer to a set dollar amount such as $10 or $15 for an office visit, rather than a percentage.)

- **Deductible.** The deductible is a set dollar amount in dental expenses that must be paid each calendar year by a consumer before the consumer is eligible for coverage. Typically, this runs around $100 or less per person covered and may exclude cleanings and x-rays.

- **Preauthorization.** This is the process whereby the dentist submits the consumer's treatment plan and x-rays to the insurance company *before* any work is done. The company and its dental consultants determine the amount it will reimburse the consumer for the work. Preauthorization is required by most plans for procedures costing more than a specified amount.

- **Schedule of benefits.** This is the list of procedures and the maximum amount the insurance company will reimburse the consumer.

- **Usual, customary and reasonable (UCR).** Based on fees charged by a sampling of dentists from the consumer's geographic region (usually by zip code), UCR is an average fee for a specified service. Insurers using UCR then apply a percentage to determine how much the insurer pays (for example, the insurer will pay 80 percent of the UCR for fillings; the consumer pays anything over that).

Traditional Indemnity Insurance

Basically, traditional indemnity insurance reimburses you or your dentist in part or in full for care provided. A claim form must be submitted to receive that payment. If your dentist agrees to accept assignment, she agrees to accept as payment in full the amount the insurance company will pay, and the check will be mailed directly to her. If your dentist does not accept assignment, you will pay her bill, submit the claim form and receive the check as reimbursement.

Indemnity insurers base their payments either on the usual, customary and reasonable (UCR) fees charged by dentists in your region or on a fixed schedule of fees for each procedure. In either case, your dentist's fees may be higher, and unless she accepts assignment, you will have to pay the difference between the insurance company's payment and your dentist's fee.

It is common for indemnity plans to pay 100 percent of the cost of preventive services such as cleanings and examinations; 80 percent of the cost of fillings and root canal therapy; 50 percent of crowns, bridges and dentures; and nothing for orthodontics or cosmetic dentistry. The percentages may vary from plan to plan, but in all cases, the balance is your coinsurance, for which you are responsible. Your dentist may need to submit a treatment plan in advance to get preauthorization for treatment in order to ensure coverage, especially for costly procedures such as the extraction of several teeth or root canals and crown placements for one or more teeth.

You may also be responsible for an annual deductible. This is a fixed, usually modest amount (around $100 or less) of your dental bill that you must pay each year before you are eligible for reimbursement of subsequent fees. In other words, the first $100 or so of each year's dental costs are not covered, except for cleaning or other preventive services.

Indemnity plans commonly have maximum levels of benefits, as well. The annual maximum sets a limit on how much will be reimbursed for the year, either for each member or for your entire family. You may also find a lifetime maximum, frequently related to orthodontic work or similar high-fee procedures.

While an indemnity plan may put limits on payments for certain types of procedures or on the amount of coverage, it does not limit your choice of dentist. Of all types of insurance, indemnity offers you the greatest freedom of choice about who provides your dental care.

Managed Care

The first dental managed care plan was created in the mid-1950s in California, but this type of plan has not become as common in dentistry as in medicine. In 1996, two-thirds of dental practices had no patients covered by managed care plans. Nevertheless, the growth rate of enrollment in managed care plans is currently greater than that in indemnity plans.

As we described in chapter 1, there are two main types of dental managed care plans: preferred provider organizations (PPOs) and health maintenance organizations (HMOs), also called capitated plans. PPOs offer consumers a list of dentists who have agreed to provide services at a discounted fee. As long as the consumer goes to one of the plan dentists, he or she receives benefits. Typically, there are no deductibles and no copayments on cleanings and other preventive services. Copayments are usually required, however, for fillings, crowns and other more expensive procedures. The consumer must submit a claim form and be reimbursed for fees. The advantage to PPOs is the discount, which varies but may be as much as 25 percent.

Consumers in HMOs must also select from a network of dentists in order to get benefits. The dentists have agreed to provide care in exchange for an amount prepaid by the insurer per consumer per month. The dentist receives this payment whether the patient visits the office or not. For the consumer, HMOs eliminate claim forms and delays in reimbursement. Preventive services are usually covered in full (some plans may have a small copayment, such as $5 or $10 per office visit); other covered services usually have a patient copayment. Most HMOs don't have annual or lifetime maximums.

Direct Reimbursement

Employers looking for ways to offer benefits to their employees while controlling costs have found an alternative to either traditional indemnity insurance or managed care. It's called direct reimbursement (DR). Its simplicity and potential for lower costs have attracted about 1,000 employers to try it. Yours may be one.

Here's how DR works. An employee covered by a direct reimbursement dental plan pays the dentist at the time services are provided—much like the traditional, fee-for-service system. The major difference is that the employee submits a claim to his or her employer for reimbursement of the payment made.

Because each DR plan is custom designed for an employer, plan details vary. However, most plans do not have deductibles or complicated fee schedules. The benefits vary, but may be structured so that all of the first $100 is covered, 80 percent of the next $100 and 50 percent of all remaining dental expenses until the maximum annual benefit of $1,200 for each person covered. Determining how much will be reimbursed tends to be straightforward and simple for both patient and dentist.

Although DR plans are not new, consumers' experience with or exposure to this type of plan is. Be especially careful before you sign up. Ask a lot of questions such as the following:

1. **Will the plan administrator be a fellow employee, with other duties that might interfere with his or her ability to pay promptly?**

2. **If the administrator is a third party, does the party have experience with similar plans for companies of similar size?**

3. **What are the specific details of the benefits?**

4. **How do benefits compare with any alternative plans?**

5. **What will the process for filing a claim be?**

6. **Who will handle inquiries or complaints about reimbursement?**

7. **Who will fund the plan—your employer, you and your fellow employees or some combination?**

8. **What happens if funding is inadequate—will additional funds be available or will you be denied benefits?**

9. **Has the company made provision for employees who are laid off to purchase benefits for a specified time period?**
   This is required by law, but you should still make sure the company has fulfilled this obligation.

With DR, you have free choice of dentist. You know what will be covered, and you'll probably receive reimbursement quickly and without hassles. Before you select a DR plan, just take the time you need to find out how your employer's particular plan will work and whether it is right for you.

Questions About Insurance Plans

If your company offers dental benefits, you will face the decision about participating in a plan at the start of your employment or when a new plan is introduced, as well as annually during a specified benefits enrollment period. Whether your choices are from among indemnity plans or managed care plans or both, read the literature from each plan carefully. Talk with your benefits manager or the dental plan representative. You will want answers to questions such as the following:

1. What services are covered?

2. Do I have a choice of dentists?

3. Are services from my current dentist covered?

4. How are referrals to specialists handled? Who pays?

5. What are my costs—a portion of the premium, deductibles, copayments, uncovered services?

6. Is there a limit, or maximum, on benefits, either annually or over a lifetime?

7. Are preexisting conditions covered?

8. What is the appeal process when coverage is denied?

9. How long has the insurer offered similar plans?

10. For plans that reimburse fees, what is the process for filing a claim? What is the average length of time for payment?

11. Are second opinions covered?

12. What mechanisms are in place for surveying patient satisfaction?

13. Is there a toll-free number for patients to call with questions or problems related to dental coverage?

Specifically for PPOs and HMOs, ask these additional questions:

1. How are dentists selected for the network?

2. Are dentists periodically evaluated by the plan?
   What is the process?

3. Under what circumstances can a dentist be removed from
   the plan? Have any been so removed?

4. How many general dentists in my area are in the network?
   How many specialists, especially periodontists and
   oral surgeons?

5. Can each member of my family have a different dentist?

6. What is the procedure for changing dentists?

7. How are emergencies handled when the network dentist's
   office is closed?

8. How is the dentist compensated?

9. Does the cost of specialty care come out of my general
   dentist's compensation?

HMOs often do this to discourage referrals to specialists. These
plans may also pay general dentists more for performing certain kinds of
specialty care such as periodontal work, which may encourage a dentist
to carry out procedures he may or may not be fully qualified to do.

If you are considering an existing plan, talk with other employees
who are enrolled in the plan. In particular, ask them:

1. Have you had any problems getting appointments when you
   wanted them?

2. How long have you usually had to wait to get an
   appointment?

3. Have you had the same dentist since you began in the plan?
   If not, why not?

4. Have the procedures you needed been covered? Have you
   ever had to appeal denial of coverage?

5. If this is a plan that reimburses for fees, how long on average
   has it taken to receive payment?

Alternatives to Employer Plans

What if your employer doesn't offer dental benefits? You may still be able to find group dental coverage with a little shopping around. Among the possible sources are:

- Labor unions
- Professional membership organizations such as the National Association of Female Executives
- Credit unions, credit card companies and banks
- Local dental society

Commonly, these plans are a version of PPO, which for an annual fee provides access to a list of dentists who have agreed to discount their services to consumers who are members of the PPO. Before you get out your checkbook to pay the annual fee, however, examine the plan and its suitability for your circumstances very carefully.

- Check to see if the finances make sense. Suppose you are single and thirty-something with healthy teeth that to date have only needed preventive visits and an occasional filling. If you join a PPO with a $75 annual fee and a 10 percent discount on services, you'll need to spend $750 a year to recoup your annual fee. That's a lot of cleanings! If the discount is 25 percent, then you'll need to spend $300 a year to recoup your annual fee.

- Find out who the network dentists are. You probably won't be able to see the entire list of network dentists without paying the annual fee, but you can ask how many are available in your area. You can also ask your current dentist if he participates. Also, make sure to ask how dentists are selected for the network and what, if any, quality controls the PPO has in place to continue evaluating participating dentists.

- Get it in writing. Don't sign up for any plan without a written description, including the discounts, fees, copayments (if any), services covered and procedures for changing dentists or canceling the plan.

- Evaluate the dentist(s). Follow the procedures described in chapter 1 for evaluating network dentists. Remember that they are receiving less income for caring for you. Does that mean that they will try to carry out more procedures, give you less desirable appointment times or otherwise give you less quality care than you deserve? That's for you to determine. Never relinquish quality for price in dental care.

When You and Your Insurer Disagree

If your insurer or managed care plan refuses to authorize treatment or to reimburse you for a claim, you should talk directly with a claims manager or supervisor. Find out exactly why the claim was denied. If the treatment plan (submitted for preauthorization) or claim form (submitted for reimbursement) was incomplete or incorrect, work with your dentist to provide the necessary information and resubmit the plan or form.

If the insurer has decided the procedure is ineligible for coverage, review your policy carefully. If you believe the procedure is in fact eligible, submit a written request for a reconsideration. Have the dentist provide x-rays, a narrative of the key points in your case and any references to the dental literature that support the narrative. Note the section of the policy under which you believe coverage is authorized.

If you are dissatisfied with the review, call your state insurance department. Ask if your state has a claims appeal process and/or arbitration panel. Follow the necessary procedures to take this step.

Finally, if you remain dissatisfied after trying all of the above and the amount in dispute is substantial, you may want to consult an attorney about filing a lawsuit.

WHEN DENTAL CARE IS NOT COVERED BY INSURANCE

In chapter 2, we described several low-cost alternatives for getting the dental care you need if you have no dental insurance and are unable to pay standard fees. These sites include government clinics, the Veterans Administration and dental school clinics. You may also find that through your local dental society, area dentists will provide care at significantly reduced fees for residents who qualify.

Even if you have dental insurance coverage, there's always the chance that you will need a procedure that is not fully covered by your plan. Orthodontics is one particularly expensive procedure frequently ignored by insurers. In fact, about half of all dental expenses are paid by consumers, without any reimbursement. What can you do if you need care for which you have little or no insurance coverage? Here are some suggestions.

■ Discuss your circumstances with your dentist when she presents the treatment plan. She may be able to suggest an alternative procedure that is less expensive or divide the work into several segments, each of which can be paid for before the next one is begun. She can also advise you on how long you could wait before having the procedure done, giving you time to save or borrow the necessary funds.

Medicare and Dentistry

If you are 65 years of age or older or meet the Social Security Administration's criteria for disability, you are eligible for Medicare. However, you probably won't be surprised to learn that your Medicare coverage provides very little in the way of dental coverage.

Among the dental procedures eligible for Medicare coverage are treatment of infections, biopsies and removal of tumors, tooth extractions necessitated by chemotherapy and hospital fees for the care of a medically compromised patient (see chapter 6) undergoing dental care. However, a 1993 survey of hospital-based dentists by the Federation of Special Care Organizations in Dentistry found that claims for procedures eligible for coverage were frequently rejected—either because the company administering the Medicare plan interpreted the eligibility rules inconsistently or wrongly or incomplete information was submitted on the claim form. When fees were reimbursed, they were on average just 33 percent of actual charges.

- Ask about available payment options. Your dentist may not advertise her willingness to provide care on an installment plan, but if you ask, she may indeed agree to weekly or monthly payments for care. She may also accept major credit cards.

- Consider getting a second opinion. It's unwise to shop for the lowest bidder without consideration of quality, but fees vary widely, even among equally qualified dentists.

- Look carefully at your automobile liability or medical insurance coverage. If dental treatment is needed as the result of an automobile accident, your automobile liability policy (in a no-fault state) or the insurer of the other vehicle may pay for the procedure. If you need to have oral surgery to remove a tumor or extract several impacted teeth, your medical insurance may cover some or all of the expenses. However, as a general rule, medical insurance provides dental benefits only when necessary for the treatment of fractures or dislocations of the jaw. Other dental services—for example, bridges, crowns and dentures—are not covered under such plans unless the procedures are necessary to maintain your dental health *as a result of a nondental medical illness or injury.*

- Examine whether you qualify for Medicaid in your state (call your state department of welfare or social services). While the federally funded, state-administered Medicaid program primarily covers medical care, you may be able to get necessary dental care. Program details vary from state to state.

No matter what improvements have been made over the years in professional dental care, your oral health is largely in your own hands. When you do consult a dentist, it must be as partners. This book was written to guide you in that partnership. You have a right to information about your oral health and any planned therapy and to competent, pain-free care. You also have a responsibility to ask questions, make informed decisions, challenge the dentist when you believe something to be wrong or amiss and carry out the dentist's instructions about home care. As partners, you and your dentist can help ensure that your teeth give you a lifetime of use.

DENTIST INFORMATION WORKSHEET

NAME OF DENTIST ▶	DENTIST 1	DENTIST 2	DENTIST 3
Is this dentist accepting new patients?			
If "no," when will he/she accept new patients?			
Does this dentist allow get-acquainted visits?			
If "yes," how much time will I be given on this visit?			
How much will it cost?			
Do patients have direct telephone access to the dentist?			
Are there specific call-in hours per week?			
If "yes," when?			
Does this dentist limit his/her practice to a specialty?			
If "yes," what specialty?			
Is this dentist board certified in his/her specialty?			
When and where did this dentist receive his/her dental training?			
Did this dentist complete a general dentistry residency?			

NAME OF DENTIST ▶	DENTIST 1	DENTIST 2	DENTIST 3
How long has this dentist been in practice?			
Has he/she ever practiced in another state?			
When does this dentist's current license to practice expire?			
Has he/she ever had a dental license suspended or revoked in this state or elsewhere?			
What procedures does this dentist commonly perform?			
Has he/she had special training to carry out procedures such as implants?			
If so, how long was it and where did he/she receive it?			
Is this dentist in a solo or group practice?			
If group, are dentists same specialty?			
If group, are dentists different specialties?			
Is there a licensed hygienist on staff?			
Does the hygienist do all the cleaning and polishing?			
Does the dentist do cleaning and polishing, on request?			
Is the dental assistant certified?			
How often do the dentist and staff attend conferences and continuing education workshops?			

continued

APPENDIX: DENTIST INFORMATION WORKSHEET *continued*

NAME OF DENTIST ▶	DENTIST 1	DENTIST 2	DENTIST 3
Who performs x-ray examinations?			
If it's someone other than the dentist, has he/she received formal training?			
Does the dentist provide a written treatment plan?			
Does it include fees?			
Does this dentist publish a list of his/her fees?			
What is the cost of a basic dental exam, cleaning and x-ray?			
What is the cost of a basic silver (amalgam) filling (one surface)?			
Is payment demanded at the time of service?			
Does this dentist permit a flexible payment schedule?			
Will my dental insurance be accepted?			
Will the dentist file all insurance claims?			
Does this dentist participate in or offer a prepaid dental plan?			
Does this dentist have hospital admitting privileges?			
If "yes," name the hospital(s).			
Is this dentist's location convenient to where I live?			
Is there adequate parking at the dentist's office?			

NAME OF DENTIST ▶	DENTIST 1	DENTIST 2	DENTIST 3
Is public transportation available to the dentist's office?			
Does this dentist have flexible office hours?			
Evening appointments?			
Weekend appointments?			
Is the reception area clean, well-lit and large enough to accommodate waiting patients and their families?			
Do people seem to wait a long time?			
Was I greeted promptly?			
Was I seen on time?			
Are current health-related reading materials available?			
Will I be given copies of my entire dental record?			
If "no," will I be given a summary of my dental records?			
Will I be given copies of my x-rays?			
If "no," will my x-rays be sent to another dentist?			
Will I be charged for this service?			
How much will it cost?			
Who covers for the dentist when he/she is ill or on vacation?			

Make additional copies of this form as needed.

GLOSSARY

Note: Words within a definition that are shown in boldface are defined elsewhere in the Glossary.

Abscess: Pus formation in the bone or soft tissue, caused by infection.

Allograft: A graft of bone tissue taken from a cadaver and implanted in a person's **alveolar bone** to fill in irregularities caused by disease or injury.

Alloplast: A graft of inert metal or plastic material implanted in a person's **alveolar bone** to fill in irregularities caused by disease or injury.

Alveolar bone: The part of the jawbone in which a tooth's root sits.

Alveolar osteitis: Infection of the **alveolar bone.**

Amalgam: A metallic alloy of silver, tin and mercury used to fill teeth; also called a silver filling.

Apicoectomy: Surgical removal of the root tip, usually to remove an area of infection.

Autograft: A graft of a person's own bone tissue, taken from the hip or **alveolar bone** and implanted in the person's alveolar bone to fill in irregularities caused by disease or injury.

Bacteremia: Bacterial infection of the bloodstream.

Behavior management: Techniques used to assure the cooperation of young patients. At least 10 are available and used by dentists when treating children, ranging from showing the child what will be done before proceeding to holding the child down.

Bicuspid: A type of **permanent tooth,** located between the pointed **canine** teeth and **molars.**

Biopsy: Surgical removal of a small amount of tissue to carry out tests to determine the types of cells present; commonly used to diagnose cancer.

Bitewing x-ray: An x-ray of the **crowns** of the upper and lower back teeth taken together to view how the teeth fit with one another and to identify possible areas of decay.

Bleaching: A cosmetic dental procedure using peroxide or other bleaching agent to remove stains from teeth.

Bonding: A cosmetic dental procedure in which the tooth is etched with acid and tooth-colored **composite resin** is applied with adhesive to change the surface or shape of a damaged tooth.

Braces: Orthodontic appliances applied to teeth to correct **malocclusion.**

Bridge: A **prosthesis** that can be either fixed or removable to replace one or a few missing teeth.

Bruxism: Grinding, clenching or gnashing of teeth.

Calculus: Plaque hardened into crusty deposits on the surface of teeth; also called tartar.

Canine: A type of **permanent tooth,** with a pointed end, located between the **incisors** and **bicuspids.**

Cantilever bridge: A **prosthesis,** used to replace one or two missing teeth, that is attached at one end to an artificial **crown** covering a remaining tooth.

Caries: Bacterial disease that causes cavities; also called decay.

Cavity: A hole in a tooth, caused by **caries.**

Cementum: The thin outermost layer covering the tooth root, to which the **periodontal ligament** attaches.

Composite resin: A plastic used to fill teeth in place of **amalgam;** also used in tooth **bonding** and as a **sealant.**

Condyle: The round end of the **mandible,** which fits into the **fossa** to form the **temporomandibular joint.**

Cosmetic dentistry: A type of dentistry that involves procedures done solely to improve appearance.

Crown: (1) The part of the tooth visible above the gum line. (2) A type of tooth restoration in which an artificial (gold or **porcelain**) tooth is placed over a badly decayed or broken tooth, retaining the natural root but entirely covering the specially prepared natural crown; also called a cap.

Dental assistant: A professional who works chairside with a dentist, setting up for procedures, handing instruments and carrying out procedures and other general assistance tasks.

Dental hygienist: A trained professional who cleans teeth, takes x-rays, carries out preliminary oral examinations and provides education on oral hygiene. State laws vary as to other tasks a hygienist may carry out, including applying **fluoride** and **sealants,** polishing teeth after the dentist applies filling material and giving a **topical anesthetic.**

Dental practice acts: The laws of a state that govern the practice of dentistry.

Dentin: The predominant material of teeth, lying under the **enamel** in the **crown** and under the **cementum** in the root.

Denture: A plastic **prosthesis** that replaces some or all of a person's teeth.

Disk: Cartilage that lies between the **condyle** and **fossa** of the **temporomandibular joint.**

Distal: The side of a tooth that is away from the midline of the face.

Enamel: The hard substance that covers the natural **crown** of a tooth.

Endodontics: The dental specialty that carries out **root canal therapy** and other treatments for diseases of the dental **pulp.**

Extraction: Removal of a tooth.

Facial: The surface of a tooth that lies against the inside of the cheek.

Fixed bridge: A **prosthesis,** used to replace one or two missing teeth, that is permanently attached at both ends to artificial **crowns** placed on remaining teeth.

Fluoridation: The process of adding **fluoride** to water supplies to help prevent tooth decay.

Fluoride: A mineral that protects teeth from decay.

Fluorosis: A brown staining of teeth, caused by too much **fluoride** in water supplies, usually from natural sources.

Fossa: The socket into which the **condyle** of the **temporomandibular joint** fits.

Full denture: A plastic **prosthesis** replacing all of a person's teeth.

General dentist: A dentist who does not specialize in any particular type of dentistry and who has not undergone advanced specialty training.

Gingiva: The tissue, commonly called gums, that covers the **alveolar bone** and surrounds each tooth.

Gingivitis: Inflammation of the **gingiva.**

Gutta percha: A rubberlike material that is used to fill the root canal during **root canal therapy,** once the nerve has been removed.

Handpiece: The dentist's drill.

Hemisection: A surgical procedure involving the removal of one or more roots and a portion of the natural **crown** from a **molar** during **root canal therapy.**

Impacted tooth: A **permanent tooth** that does not erupt into its normal position but remains fully or partially embedded in the bone.

Implant: A surgical procedure in which a metal framework, post or blade is inserted under the gum tissue and/or into the **alveolar bone** to provide a means of attaching a **crown, bridge** or **denture.**

Impression: An imprint of some or all of the mouth, made in a soft material from which a **study cast** is made; used in preparing **crowns, bridges** and **dentures.**

Incisor: A type of **permanent tooth** located in the front of the mouth, between the two **canine** teeth.

Jaw dysfunction: Abnormal operation of the **temporomandibular joint.** An example is the inability of the jaw to open fully.

Lingual: The surface of a tooth that faces the tongue.

Maintenance visit: A visit to the dentist for **prophylaxis** and examination, usually on a semiannual or annual basis; also called a recall visit.

Malocclusion: A bad bite caused by the upper and lower teeth not meeting properly when they are brought together.

Mandible: The lower jawbone that contains the lower teeth.

Maryland bridge: A **prosthesis,** used to replace one or two missing teeth, that is attached to the surface of the remaining teeth on either side.

Maxilla: The upper jawbone that contains the upper teeth.

Medically compromised: People who have chronic medical conditions or illnesses that require special care to prevent infection or other complications when undergoing dental treatment.

Mesial: The surface of a tooth that faces toward the midline of the face.

Molar: A type of tooth, located in the back of the mouth, behind the **bicuspids.**

Mucosa: The tissue that lines the inside of the mouth and covers the tongue.

Nitrous oxide: A gas inhaled to reduce anxiety and awareness of pain in dental patients; also called laughing gas.

Occlusal: The biting or chewing surface of a tooth.

Operatory: A dental treatment room.

Oral and maxillofacial surgery: The dental specialty that involves surgery to the jaw, mouth and related muscles, including tooth extraction; also called oral surgery.

Oral pathology: The dental specialty that deals with the diagnosis of diseases of the mouth using **biopsy** and other testing techniques.

Orthodontics: The dental specialty that uses **braces** and other orthodontic appliances to correct **malocclusion.**

Osseointegration: The natural process whereby jawbone tissue grows snugly against a metallic **implant** to help ensure a secure attachment.

Overdenture: A removable **denture** that clips onto an **implant** at the front of the mouth, resting on the gum and jaw in the rest of the mouth.

Palate: The roof of the mouth.

Partial denture: A removable **prosthesis,** used to replace a few missing teeth, that uses a metal framework and clasps to attach the prosthesis to adjoining teeth.

Pediatric dentistry: The dental specialty that provides dental care to children; also called pedodontics.

Periapical x-ray: An x-ray that shows a tooth's **crown,** root and surrounding bone structure.

Periodontal disease: Inflammation and degeneration of the gum tissue surrounding the teeth and covering the **alveolar bone;** also called periodontitis.

Periodontal ligament: The strong fibers that surround the root of a tooth and attach it to the **alveolar bone.**

Periodontics: The dental specialty that treats **periodontal disease.**

Permanent teeth: The adult teeth, usually 32 in number.

Plaque: A deposit of material on the tooth surface that harbors bacteria and acid formation, causing tooth decay.

Porcelain: A hard, tooth-colored substance used to make artificial **crowns,** especially in highly visible parts of the mouth where a natural appearance is important.

Primary teeth: A child's first teeth; also called baby or deciduous teeth.

Prophylaxis: Professional cleaning of teeth to remove stains, **calculus** and **plaque.**

Prosthesis: An artificial appliance created to replace missing teeth or to restore a damaged part of the mouth.

Prosthodontics: The dental specialty that provides replacements for missing teeth or damage to the jaw or mouth.

Public health dentistry: The dental specialty that carries out programs on community dental education, community/school dental screening and **fluoridation** information.

Pulp: Cells, fibers, blood vessels and nerves contained in the root canal, which runs through the tooth's **crown** and root.

Resorption: A natural process involving the dissolving of **alveolar bone,** roots or **dentin** as the result of disease or abnormal pressure.

Restoration: A filling, **crown, bridge** or **denture** that replaces lost tooth structure or an entire tooth.

Root canal therapy: A dental procedure in which the **pulp** is removed from the root canal, which is cleaned, filled with **gutta percha** and sealed prior to placing a **crown** or filling.

Root planing: A technique of **prophylaxis** involving the scraping of the root surface below the gum line to remove **plaque** and **calculus.**

Saliva: The clear secretion of the salivary glands into the mouth.

Scaling: A technique of **prophylaxis** involving the scraping of the crown surface to remove stains, **plaque** and **calculus** from a tooth.

Sealant: A **composite resin** substance applied to the pits and fissures of teeth, especially **molars,** to protect them from decay.

Splint: A device, usually removable, designed to reinforce or protect teeth. An example is a bite guard put in the mouth at night to prevent **bruxism.**

Stomatitis: Inflammation of the oral **mucosa.**

Study cast: Plaster cast made from an **impression** of a person's teeth and/or gums, used to plan oral surgery, **implant** placement, jaw realignment, the fabrication of **dentures** and other procedures requiring a duplicate of the person's mouth.

Temporomandibular disorders: A group of conditions involving the **temporomandibular joint** that include symptoms of facial or jaw pain, headaches and **jaw dysfunction.**

Temporomandibular joint: The joint that connects the jawbone to the skull near the ear.

Third molar: The **molar** farthest back in the mouth, the last **permanent tooth** to erupt; also called a wisdom tooth.

Topical anesthetic: A medication applied by spraying or swabbing the gum surface to lessen the pain of an oral injection.

Topical fluoride: The application of a solution or gel containing **fluoride** to the outer surfaces of the teeth.

Transcutaneous electric nerve stimulation (TENS): A method of pain control that uses electric signals sent to nerve endings.

Universal precautions: Part of the infection control procedures used by dental workers to protect patients and themselves from infections, including wearing face masks and eye protection, latex gloves and clean, protective clothing.

Veneer: A cosmetic facing that attaches to the outer surface of a tooth with adhesive.

Xerostomia: A condition caused by inadequate production of **saliva** by the salivary glands; also called dry mouth.

SUGGESTED READING

Christensen, Gordon J. *A Consumer's Guide to Dentistry.* St. Louis, Mo.: Mosby, 1994.

Friedman, Jay W., and the Editors of Consumer Reports Books. *Complete Guide to Dental Health.* Yonkers, N.Y.: Consumer Reports Books, 1991.

Kaplan, S.D.B. *Everything the Dental Patient Always Wanted to Know, but Was Afraid to Ask.* New York: Smithtown Dental Book Co., 1987.

Klatell, Jack, Andrew Kaplan, and Gray Williams, Jr. *The Mount Sinai Medical Center Family Guide to Dental Health.* New York: Macmillan, 1991.

Linkow, Leonard I. *Without Dentures: The Miracle of Dental Implants.* Hollywood, Fla.: Frederick Fell Publishers, 1987.

Stay, Flora Parsa. *The Complete Book of Dental Remedies.* Garden City Park, N.Y.: Avery, 1996.

Taintor, Jerry F. *The Oral Report: The Consumer's Commonsense Guide to Better Dental Care.* New York: Facts on File, 1988.

INDEX

Surface electromyograph (EMG), 202
Surfaces of tooth, 118
Surgery. *See* Oral surgery; *specific types*

T

Teaching hospitals, 73, 76-77
Teeth
    anatomy of, 117
    baby, 142
    bleaching, 208-209
    bonding, 209
    brushing, 120, 159, 172
    cleaning
        in bacteria control, 174
        by dental hygienists, 31
        in child dental care, 140
        in dentist's office visit, 98-101
        oral prophylaxis, 98
        in preventive dental care, 98-101
    clenching, 200
    crooked and misaligned, 158-159, 178
    decay of, 120, 124-125, 171
    extraction of, 131-135, 183
    flossing, 120, 159, 172
    grinding, 118, 200, 204
    impacted, 131, 133
    missing, replacement of, 178-180
    permanent, 116
    polishing, 99
    primary, 142
    protecting
        with fluoride treatment, 146-148
        with sealant, 149-150
    repair and restoration of
        crowns, 125-127, 141
        fillings, 121-125
        root canal therapy, 125, 127-130
    surfaces of, 118
    types of, 115-118
    whitening, 208-209
    wisdom, 116, 130, 132
Tell-show-do behavior management, 151
Temporal bone, 196
Temporary health conditions, 187
Temporomandibular disorder (TMD)
    American Dental Association and, 196
    diagnosis of, 198-203
    incidence of, 198
    symptoms of, 90, 92, 195-198
    treatment of
        nonsurgical, 203-205
        surgical, 205-207
Temporomandibular joint disorder (TMJ).
    See Temporomandibular disorder
Temporomandibular (TM) joint, 196
TENS, 192, 204
Testing, dental education and licensing,
    36, 39, 40, 45, 66
    radiography, 66
Tetracycline, 208
Third molars, 116, 130, 132
Thrush (fungus), 119
Titanium dental implants, 212
TMD. *See* Temporomandibular disorder
TMJ. *See* Temporomandibular disorder
Tongue braces, 159-160
Tongue tumors, 119-120
Tools, dental, 92
Topical anesthetics, 104
Topical fluoride, 99, 148
Tranquilizers, 108. *See also* Sedatives
Transcutaneous electric nerve stimulation
    (TENS), 192, 204
Transosteal dental implant, 212-213
Treatment, dental
    in child dental care
        behavior management, 150-153
        general anesthesia, 153-158
        orthodontics, 158-161
        pain control, 153-158
        sedatives, 151, 153-158
    dental conditions needing, 119-120
    disagreements about, 35-36
    in elderly dental care
        dentures, 180-181
        missing teeth replacement, 178-180
        periodontal disease, 171-172, 174-178
    mouth and, anatomy of, 115-118
    oral surgery, 135-137
    patient-dentist relationship in, 16-17,
        24, 115
    plan, preventive dental care and, 97-98
    refusal of, right to, 164-166
    temporomandibular disorder
        nonsurgical, 203-205
        surgical, 205-207
    tooth extraction, 131-135
    tooth repair and restoration
        crowns, 125-127, 129, 141, 217
        fillings, 121-125
        root canal therapy, 125, 127-130
    variations in, 16